Learning Biochemistry

100 CASE ORIENTED PROBLEMS

Learning Biochemistry

100 CASE ORIENTED PROBLEMS

Richard F. Lalueña

Department of Biochemistry
The University of Texas Health Science Center
San Antonio, Texas

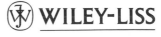 **WILEY-LISS**

A JOHN WILEY & SONS, INC. , PUBLICATION
NEW YORK • CHICHESTER • BRISBANE • TORONTO • SINGAPORE

Address All Inquiries to the Publisher
Wiley-Liss, Inc., 605 Third Avenue, New York, NY 10158-0012

Library of Congress Cataloging-in-Publication Data
Ludueña, Richard F.
  Learning biochemistry : 100 case oriented problems / Richard F.
Ludueña.
      p.   cm.
  Includes bibliographical references and index.
  ISBN 0-471-01887-2
  1. Clinical biochemistry—Problems, exercises, etc.   I. Title.
RB112.5.L83   1994
616.07'076—dc20   94-43218
                                                                         CIP

The text of this book is printed on acid-free paper.

10 9 8 7 6 5 4 3 2 1

To my students

Contents

CONTENTS

Preface

Many people have helped in the preparation of this book. The staff of the Dolph Briscoe Library at the University of Texas Health Science Center at San Antonio have been very helpful in providing assistance with Plusnet. To Drs. Martin Adamo, Jeff Hansen, John Lee, Fredrik Leeb-Lundberg, Bettie Sue Masters, and Barry Nall, my colleagues in teaching the Medical Biochemistry course, a heartfelt thanks for their support, encouragement, and helpful comments, and particular thanks to Dr. Merle Olson, who is both my teaching colleague and my chairman, for his assistance. I thank Dr. Lois Bready of the University of Texas Health Science Center at San Antonio and Dr. Marc Fellous of the Institut Pasteur for suggesting problems and Dr. David Williams of the University of Toronto for permitting me to use some unpublished information. I would like to acknowledge Dr. William Curtis, of Wiley-Liss, my editor, whose encouragement and commonsense suggestions have been very valuable and saved much time. Despite the assistance all these people have provided, all the mistakes here are my own.

A very special thank you to my wife, Linda, and daughter, Sara, not only for their loving support, but for putting up with my distraction and my pounding on the computer keyboard in the small hours of the morning. For analogous patience, I would like to thank the people in my laboratory, particularly Mary Carmen Roach, for locating the Chemintosh program used to prepare the illustrations.

Finally, I would like to thank the 17 classes of medical students who have made teaching them such a pleasure as well as a challenge and whose needs, as I perceived them, led to the creation of this book. These problems have been refined and improved by being tested first on the classes entering in 1991, 1992, and 1993. In honor of their support and hard work, this book is dedicated to them.

Introduction for
the Professor

Genesis

I have had the pleasure and privilege of teaching medical students for the last 17 years. Although I enjoy lecturing very much, I recognize that there are limitations to the lecture system. In many ways it is a passive system of learning in which the professor expounds and the student memorizes. The syllabus and the text are in essence aids to memory. The examinations are in large part assays to measure the extent of memorization that has occurred. In this system the students take little responsibility for their own learning. Their questions are often driven by the desire to delineate with the highest possible exactitude the precise boundary between what is and what is not required to be committed to memory. In the scramble for grades, the beauty of biochemistry is easy to miss. Even if that beauty animates the lecturer, there may not be enough time to have it illuminate a great deal of the course content. Often, even in medical biochemistry, there is little time to expand on clinical applications of the corpus of information. This is unfortunate because, after all, the students are in medical school to learn how to treat patients; they want to see how biochemistry relates to real patients. Often, students resent what they perceive as a lack of "relevance." That is not to say that a medical biochemistry course has no clinical relevance. There is usually enough time to tell students about the biochemical basis of diabetes, hemophilia, and a few other diseases. There are, of course, a whole host of other clinically relevant topics that could be discussed were there time enough.

The size of the typical medical class makes it difficult to address some of these problems. When you lecture to 200 students, how can you relate to each one individually and talk to them about the aspects of biochemistry that interest them? For all of these reasons, there has recently been a movement to drop lectures in favor of small-group discussions and problem-based learning. Although these are excellent formats for learning, there are formidable logistical problems to overcome to restructure a curriculum in this fashion. I thought that it would be good to have a vehicle that could add a dimension of problem-based learning to a lecture-centered course or which could be used in small-group discussions in a nontraditional curriculum. I conceived of this venture as one that would add flexibility to the curriculum.

I created these library projects about three years ago. I made up about 230 problems, from which I have chosen 100 for this book. I wanted to oblige the students to use the library as a resource where information could be found. Naturally, I had to choose problems whose answers could not be deduced from the rest of the course material: namely, the textbook, the syllabus, or the lectures. For this reason you will not see any problems about diseases such as diabetes or classic hemophilia, whose etiology is discussed in most biochemistry textbooks. Our textbook is Devlin's *Textbook of Biochemistry with Clinical Correlations*, 3rd edition. As its name implies, this is a textbook with numerous clinical correlations; it discusses the biochemical bases of quite a few diseases. For the problems in this book, therefore, I have had to find other diseases, not discussed in Devlin's book. In a sense, this book is constructed around that text and is complementary to it. However, this book could be used just as easily to accompany any other biochemistry textbook.

I have assigned each problem to a pair of students at the beginning of the course and given them the rest of the semester to come up with the answer. Successful completion of the problem is worth 4 percentage points, added to the average of their scores on the three formal examinations. The problems are voluntary. Each year 98% of the students have chosen to do the problems. They have been very well received, with 58% of the students rating them as "very educational" and 31% as "somewhat educational." Fewer than 4% of the students rated them negatively. There have even been students who have asked to do extra problems for no extra credit.

The students are advised to show me the answers before turning them in. If they are incorrect or incomplete, I will not accept them. I will not tell them the answer, but I will point out how their answer contradicts the given facts. I ask them questions to get their thinking moving in a new direction. By this method, I get to interact one-on-one or one-on-two with about 80% of the students, thereby addressing the impersonal aspect of medical school referred to above. I might add that one of the greatest benefits that I have found in using these problems is that I get to know the majority of the students. This allows me to keep my finger on the pulse of the class and gives a very human face to the course. I can get a sense of each student's potential and personality.

Format

The format of this book is as follows. There are 100 numbered problems, covering many different areas of biochemistry. Each problem describes some kind of clinical situation, including the symptoms and some biochemical findings. These are followed by some short questions or problems, such as "What is the defective enzyme?" and "Write out the pathway in which this enzyme occurs" or "How do the symptoms arise?" or "How would you treat this patient?" At first glance some of the questions will seem very easy and some very hard. It is true that they are not of equal difficulty. However, three years of experience have shown me that my predictions as to which problems would be hard and which would be easy were way off target. Even the "easy" questions will require a trip to the library to answer. The process of researching the answer will be a serious learning experience for students. A few of the more difficult problems will require some elaborate reasoning by students. Occasionally, a hint is given in the form of a clue or even a reference to a paper to look up, but looking up this paper will not by itself solve the entire problem for students but rather help them narrow down what they are to look for or think about. The reasoning required by the questions is intended to exemplify and reinforce basic biochemical principles involving, for example, metabolic pathways, protein–ligand interactions, protein structure, and the genetic code. Students are expected to answer the questions briefly.

You may be worried that the "hard" questions are too hard. Rest assured that they are not. Do not think of these as test questions for which students have to carry the answers around in their heads; these are library projects. A trip to the library will fairly easily turn up the beginnings of each answer. The hardest parts of the questions are often the ones that you as professor would think are the easiest, because they require reasoning and relatively little information; for instance, if a disease involving a flavin-bound enzyme can be cured by increasing dietary flavin, the reason probably is that the defect involves the affinity of the enzyme for the flavin. This is an answer that is attainable by reasoning. Often, first-year students lack self-confidence in their ability to reason things out and turn instinctively to an authority, such as a book or other publication, to solve the problem. It is very good discipline for them to develop confidence in their own ability to think.

The book begins with a sample problem about phenylketonuria. This is intended to show students what is expected of them. The sample problem is followed by the answer, including the reasoning that led to the answer. How much of the reasoning students will be required to show in their answers to these questions is up to the professor. I describe the reasoning to show students the basic strategy for answering these questions. There follow the 100 problems themselves, each group of problems being accompanied by their answers. You could photocopy a question and give it to students or use the question and its answer as the basis of a discussion. In many cases I have made the answers quite detailed, more so than is called for by the question. This will give you more latitude in judging student responses. Some students will answer the bare minimum; others will write volumes. Although students are not asked to name the disease, if the disease has a specific name, this is given in capitals at the end of the answer.

Where are the answers to be found? The students should go to the library and browse through texts or use computerized databases. Sometimes looking up the appropriate subject in the card catalog will lead them to the answers. Some of the problems are based on the very latest findings reported in the literature, so a computerized database will be necessary. Each problem is followed by a list of references that can be consulted for further information. If you have any suggestions or corrections about the problems, I would be very grateful if you would inform me.

Some of these problems are based on very rare diseases. You may worry, as I have, that students will object that you are asking them to waste their time on a disease that has been observed in only one or two patients. So far, no student has voiced this to me as an objection, but I have two answers ready. First, students will graduate as "doctors of medicine," not as "doctors of medicine specializing in common ailments." All diseases should be within the purview of a physician, not in the absurdly impractical sense that he should know all about them, but in the sense that he should be able to search, find, and understand information about them if they should happen to turn up. Second, and more important, these questions are not intended primarily to teach students about diseases but rather, to teach them some biochemistry in an interesting and even exciting fashion and to show them that biochemistry is indeed relevant to medicine.

Administration

How the professor will use this book is entirely up to him or her. Here are some options to consider. At the beginning of the course, each student or group of students is assigned a certain number of problems. They could then turn in the problems with the answers at the end of the semester. They would be encouraged to work together, either in combinations assigned by the professor or in any fashion they desire. Their efforts will be graded and partial credit is encouraged; the scores they receive on these problems could count as a bonus, as an essential part of their grade, or as some combination of both. The problems could be discussed in conference sections, with the idea that the professor would not tell them the answers but rather, ask leading questions that could give the students an idea of where to look for the clues they need to get the answer. Students who turn in a sincere effort would get to see the answer to their questions. I would recommend not giving the answers to students who make no effort to find them out for themselves.

Of course, if enough students get to see the answers, what do you do for next year? This should not be a problem, since every week there appear in the literature new findings from which more problems such as these can be constructed. I intend to continue to do so.

In summary, this book is aimed at first-year medical students who are taking biochemistry and is intended to serve several purposes: to show students that biochemistry is indeed relevant to clinical medicine, to oblige students to take responsibility for their learning, and to teach students how to use the facilities of the library: general and specific reference books, the card catalog, computerized databases, and others. Finally, the problems are intended to be fun. If students have even half as much fun working on the problems as I did in creating them, this will have been a successful venture.

Introduction for the Student

This book contains 100 library projects in clinical biochemistry. Your professor will assign you one or more of these projects. Almost every one introduces a hypothetical patient or patients. A very brief account of the symptoms is followed by biochemical information in the form of an assay you may perform on a biopsy sample from your patient. Some questions also give you the sequence of a gene or a protein that may be altered in your patient. You are then asked various questions, such as to identify the defective enzyme, describe the metabolic pathway to which the enzyme belongs, and perhaps, to explain how the altered gene causes a defect in the enzyme or how the defective enzyme causes the symptoms. Keep in mind that in these problems, you are given the sequence of the "sense" strand of DNA. Unless otherwise indicated, all DNA sequences in this book are written in the 5'-to-3' direction.

The answers to these questions are not in your textbook or your syllabus. They will not be covered in class. To find the answers you will have to use the resources of your library. This will be excellent practice for later in medical school, when you will have to do research in the library in regard to specific patients. Look at the computerized databases in your library. The problem will give you some key words that may be useful for this search. You may also want to use the card catalog. For some problems your library may have a book that will give you the answer.

Keep in mind that looking up the problem in a book is only part of what you need to do to answer these questions. You will also have to think and use your judgment. Just because you find an answer in a book does not mean that the answer is correct. You may have found a book that is 30 years old and out of date. In general, go for the more recently published information. Remember that when you go to the library to learn more about your real patient's disease, the bottom line is to find the best information possible. If two sources contradict each other, you will have to use your judgment to decide which is more likely to be correct. You will have to reason out part of the answers to these questions using many of the basic biochemical principles you will be learning in your course. For example, when you were told that proline cannot be in an α-helix, you probably wondered what that nugget of wisdom had to do with a real patient. Some of these problems will demonstrate the connection as you use that piece of information to reason out how your patient's symptoms arise. Some questions will ask you to speculate. You will have to take your best guess, based on what you turned up in the library and what you have already reasoned out from basic principles. Do not be afraid to speculate; in the future, you will often have to do just that, deciding on the most likely course of action based on your experience and intelligence.

A sample question is provided here, based on phenylketonuria. In this question you will see what you could look up and how you would apply basic biochemical principles to solving the problem. There is also some speculation required. These questions are intended to show you the relevance of biochemistry to clinical medicine, that many diseases have a biochemical foundation, and that understanding that foundation will help you understand the disease. Another aim of the questions is to make you familiar with the library and its resources. Still another is to help you develop confidence in your own thinking. Finally, based on my years on the admissions committee, I could predict that one thing that attracted you to medical school was the intellectual challenge; these problems are intended to provide some of that challenge and to be fun. I hope that you will enjoy them as much as I have.

Sample Question

Your patient is a 2-week-old child with elevated levels of phenylpyruvic acid, phenyllactic acid, and phenylacetic acid in his urine. He has elevated levels of phenylalanine in his blood. You do a liver biopsy and prepare a cell-free extract from the liver cells. To this you add tetrahydrobiopterin and radioactive phenylalanine and find that the production of radioactive tyrosine is only 1% of that which you would expect in the case of a normal person.

a. Name the defective enzyme.

b. Write out the reaction catalyzed by the defective enzyme.

c. How would you treat this patient?

d. Assume that you have identified the defective enzyme. Assume that you have a polyclonal antibody to that enzyme from normal persons. Using the antibody, you find no evidence that the enzyme is expressed in liver cells; in a liver cell from a normal person, however, the antibody would show that the enzyme was expressed. Assume that you know the sequence of the gene coding for the enzyme in a normal person and also the sequence of the gene in your patient. Here is a portion of the gene sequence:

```
Codon number    309   310   311   312
Normal person:  GCC   TCT   CTG   GGT
Your patient:   GCC   TCT   CCG   GGT
```

Speculate on how the observed change could lead to the missing enzyme.

Answer

a. The elevated levels of phenylpyruvic acid, phenyllactic acid, and phenylacetic acid in the urine and the elevated level of phenylalanine in the blood indicate that there is a metabolic blockage somewhere. If there are abnormalities in both the blood and the urine, it is best to focus, at least initially, on the abnormality in the blood and ask "What could cause a buildup of phenylalanine?" If you look up phenylalanine metabolism in any biochemistry book, you will find that it is converted to tyrosine by the enzyme phenylalanine hydroxylase. For further information, you could look up phenylalanine hydroxylase in a computerized database. The information from the cell-free system you prepared from the liver biopsy tells you that radioactive phenylalanine is not converted to radioactive tyrosine in your patient; in other words, the defective reaction must be the one catalyzed by *phenylalanine hydroxylase.* Is it the enzyme itself that is defective, however? As any recent biochemistry book or relevant article can tell you, this particular reaction requires a cofactor called tetrahydrobiopterin. Could there be a defect in the synthesis of this cofactor? In principle, either the enzyme itself could be defective or the cofactor could be missing. However, the question tells you that in the liver cell assay you added tetrahydrobiopterin and the reaction still did not go. If the defect had been in the cofactor, addition of the cofactor would have corrected the problem, and it did not. Therefore, the defective enzyme must be phenylalanine hydroxylase.

Note: Hyperphenylalaninemia can arise secondarily to other diseases, but when you work your problems, you should assume that the answer is the simplest one that is consistent with the information given in the question.

b. Write out the reaction catalyzed by the defective enzyme.

Phenylalanine + O_2 + tetrahydrobiopterin → tyrosine + H_2O + dihydrobiopterin

Once you have identified the defective enzyme, it is very easy to find the reaction or the pathway.

c. This is not something that you need to look up. Phenylalanine is an essential amino acid. That means that we do not make it ourselves and have to have it in our diet. Normally, we would eat more phenylalanine than we really need. In a normal person, that would cause no problem, but in someone who is unable to dispose of excess phenylalanine by converting it to tyrosine, any excess phenylalanine will cause problems, including severe mental retardation, if allowed to persist. Therefore, the child should be put on a low-phenylalanine diet. The diet should have some phenylalanine since this is an essential amino acid, but the amount should be low.

d. You do not need to look up anything for this. It can be reasoned out based on information that you will learn in class. First, convert the DNA sequences to the mRNA sequences. Assume that the DNA sequence is that of the "sense" strand. To get the mRNA sequence, all you have to do is convert T to U. Then use the genetic code to derive the amino acid sequences of the normal and altered proteins. Here are the results:

Codon number	309	310	311	312
Normal person:				
DNA:	GCC	TCT	CTG	GGT
RNA:	GCC	UCU	CUG	GGU
Protein:	Ala	Ser	Leu	Gly
Your patient:				
DNA:	GCC	TCT	CCG	GGT
RNA:	GCC	UCU	CCG	GGU
Protein:	Ala	Ser	Pro	Gly

Clearly, your patient's enzyme has a proline at position 311 where the normal enzyme has a leucine. This type of mutation in which one amino acid is replaced by another is called a *missense* mutation. What effect is that likely to have on the protein? Proline is an amino acid that cannot fit into α-helices. If the normal enzyme has an α-helix that includes position 311 (we do not know that it does—that is why this is a speculation), that α-helix would be disrupted. That alone could easily wipe out the enzymatic activity of the protein, but the question tells you something else. The question tells you that *the antibody cannot detect the presence of the protein in your patient's liver cells.* With most missense mutations, the protein is still present even if it is nonfunctional and is still able to be detected by antibodies. What could cause the lack of detection? There are only two possibilities. One is that the change in conformation that results from disruption of an α-helix could destroy the antibody binding site. This possibility would have to be considered if the antibody were monoclonal, but the question describes the antibody as polyclonal, which means that it is a mixture of an enormous number of different types of antibody molecules, each type binding to the protein at a different site. It is unlikely that any conformational change would affect all possible antibody binding sites. Therefore, we are left with the other possibility, which is that the disruption of the α-helix makes the protein very unstable and causes it to be degraded by the cell's own proteolytic enzymes. Hence the enzyme is not present to react with antibodies and is not present to carry out the reaction.

Your patient has **PHENYLKETONURIA.**

References

Lichter-Konecki, U., Konecki, D. S., DiLella, A. G., Brayton, K., Marvit, J., Hahn, T. M., Trefz, F. K., and Woo, S. L. Phenylalanine hydroxylase deficiency caused by a single base substitution in an exon of the human phenylalanine hydroxylase gene. *Biochemistry* 27: 2881, 1988.

CHAPTER 1

Amino Acids

Problem 1

Your patient was born with elevated phenylalanine in his blood. To control hyperphenylalanemia, he was put on a low-phenylalanine diet. For the next 7 months, his serum phenylalanine remained very low and his mental development appeared to be normal. At 7 months, he started to have seizures and appeared to be delayed in his mental development. When he was challenged by being put briefly on a normal diet, his serum phenylalanine levels increased to well above normal. A biopsy sample was taken from his liver and treated with [^{14}C]phenylalanine in the presence of tetrahydrobiopterin. Production of [^{14}C]tyrosine was considerably higher than that observed in comparable samples from infants who had a deficiency in phenylalanine hydroxylase. A liver biopsy sample was treated with NADH and quinonoid dihydrobiopterin and the disappearance of NADH was measured spectrophotometrically. Whereas in a liver biopsy sample from a normal patient, the NADH would disappear, no loss of NADH was noted in the biopsy sample from your patient. You do one more assay in which you add NADPH and 7,8-dihydrobiopterin to the biopsy sample and measure the disappearance of NADPH; you find that this is normal.

    a. What is the defective enzyme?

    b. Write out the reaction catalyzed by the defective enzyme.

    c. Write out the pathway for biosynthesis of the cofactor.

    d. Why would he have neurologic symptoms even though he is on a low-phenylalanine diet?

Problem 2

Your patient has been blind since he was 25, shortly after immigrating here from Beirut, Lebanon. Blindness was preceded by a slow and progressive loss of vision. There is an abnormally very high concentration of ornithine in his urine. There is a slight increase in the excretion of arginine as well. Ammonia levels are normal after eating. Assume that you have identified the defective enzyme, you clone its cDNA and sequence it. The first part of the sequence (starting at the 5' end) is shown below and compared with that of the cDNA of the same enzyme obtained from a normal person. The sequence given for the normal person begins in the 5'-untranslated region and includes some of the open reading frame.

Your patient:	GAATTCCGCTGTCAGATCTGTGGTT
	TTTCTACTTGAAGGACACAATATTT
	TCCAAACTAGCACATTTGCAGAGG
Normal person:	GAATTCCGCTGTCAGATCTGTGGTT
	TTTCTACTTGAAGGACACAATGTTT
	TCCAAACTAGCACATTTGCAGAGG

a. What enzyme is your patient lacking?

b. Would you expect your patient's level of Δ^1-pyrroline 5-carboxylate to be high, low, or normal? Explain your answer. Include a diagram of the pathways involved.

c. Explain the molecular nature of the defect in the protein.

Problem 3

Your patient is a mentally retarded girl with cerebellar problems (poor coordination, slurred speech). She has abnormally high levels of succinic semialdehyde and 4-hydroxybutyrate in her urine.

    a. Which enzyme is deficient in this patient?

    b. Write out the pathway in which this enzyme occurs.

Problem 4

Your patient is a 10-month-old boy whose urine is blue. You find that the blue color follows the administration of oral tryptophan. His serum levels of tryptophan are very low. His urinary levels of tryptophan are also low.

a. What is your patient's defect?

b. When you analyze the blue pigment in his urine, you find out that it is indigo blue. How does this get made? (Write out a pathway.) (*Hint:* Think bacteria.)

Problem 5

Your patient is a 10-year-old boy who exhibits psychotic behavior and develops a rash when he is exposed to light; he also has frequent diarrhea. The symptoms appear to resemble pellagra. The level of nicotinamide in his blood is low. Although he has a normal diet, his symptoms improve greatly when you treat him with nicotinamide. His urinary and fecal levels of alanine, asparagine, glutamine, histidine, isoleucine, leucine, phenylalanine, serine, threonine, tryptophan, tyrosine, and valine are high. His blood levels of these amino acids are low. He also has high urinary and fecal levels of indoles not normally made by human enzymes.

a. Which protein is likely to be defective in your patient? In which organs would you expect the defective protein to be located?

b. How do you account for the low levels of nicotinamide in his blood? Show the pathway by which we synthesize nicotinamide.

Problem 6

Your patient is essentially symptom-free. As part of a routine check, you notice that he has elevated urinary levels of glycine, proline, and hydroxyproline. No other amino acid is elevated in the urine. Blood levels of all amino acids are normal. Studies on the family show that the elevation of these amino acids is an autosomal recessive trait.

    a. What protein is defective in your patient? In which organ is this protein located?

    b. If you have a second patient who you know is homozygous for this defect but whose urinary levels of glycine, proline, and hydroxyproline are less elevated than in the first patient, how would you characterize the difference between the defective protein of the two patients? Do not invoke a second protein.

    c. Why is your patient essentially symptom-free?

Problem 7

Your patient suffers from chronic ulcerative dermatitis and is also mentally retarded. There are high levels in his urine of dipeptides with proline as the carboxy-terminal residue. You do a biopsy and culture his fibroblasts. You prepare a cell-free extract and add the dipeptide glycylproline. You find that cleavage of the dipeptide is about 1% of that in a normal person. You culture some of your patient's fibroblasts and study them. You find that their proline levels are very low and their hydroxyproline levels are very high.

a. What is the defective enzyme? Describe the reaction that it catalyzes.

b. Speculate on how this enzyme defect could cause ulcerative dermatitis in your patient.

Problem 8

Your patient is an albino with hair that has been white from birth. He has severe vision problems. You do a karyotype on your patient and find that his chromosomes appear normal. You do a skin biopsy on your patient and culture his melanocytes. You add radioactive tyrosine to the melanocytes and find that the production of radioactive melanin is 1% of that of a normal person. You prepare a cell-free extract from the melanocytes and add radioactive tyrosine; melanin production is normal. Extensive analysis shows that your patient is lacking a protein with 12 hydrophobic domains present in normal persons.

a. What is the role of the missing protein, and how does lack of the protein cause disease in your patient?

b. You have another patient who has the same symptoms and the same biochemical findings but whose karyotype analysis reveals is missing a portion of chromosome 15. What does this tell you?

Answer 1

a. The child clearly is unable to metabolize phenylalanine. Other than being incorporated into proteins, the chief metabolic fate of phenylalanine is to be converted into tyrosine. If phenylalanine is high in the child, there must be a defect in that conversion, which is catalyzed by the enzyme *phenylalanine hydroxylase*. This enzyme requires the cofactor tetrahydrobiopterin. The fact that when tetrahydrobiopterin is present, enzyme activity is normal suggests that the defect is in the biosynthesis of the tetrahydrobiopterin cofactor rather than in the enzyme phenylalanine hydroxylase. Tetrahydrobiopterin can be formed by any one of four enzymes: (1) *sepiapterin reductase,* (2) *6-lactoyltetrahydropterin reductase,* (3) *dihydrofolate reductase,* and (4) *dihydropteridine reductase.* The first and second enzymes have as substrates sepiapterin and 6-lactoyltetrahydropterin, respectively. The third enzyme synthesizes tetrahydrobiopterin from 7,8-dihydrobiopterin and NADPH; the last assay you did shows that this process is normal in your patient. The fourth enzyme uses as its substrate quinonoid dihydrobiopterin. Since this is the substrate that in the biopsy sample is unable to be converted into tetrahydrobiopterin, this suggests that the defective enzyme is *dihydropteridine reductase.*

b. See Figure A1-1.

c. See Figure A1-2.

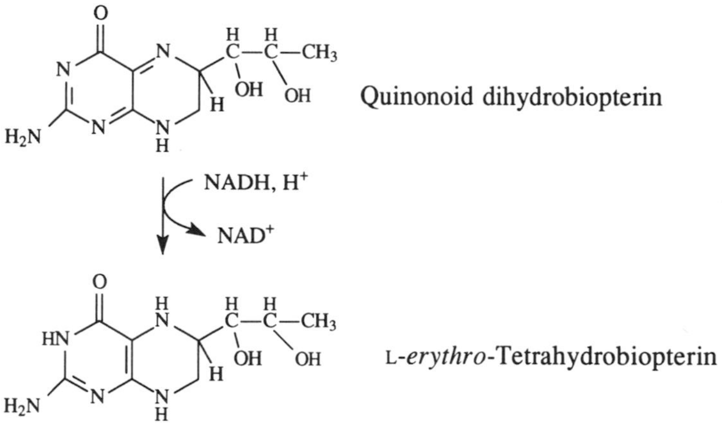

FIGURE A1-1. **Reaction catalyzed by dihydropteridine reductase.**

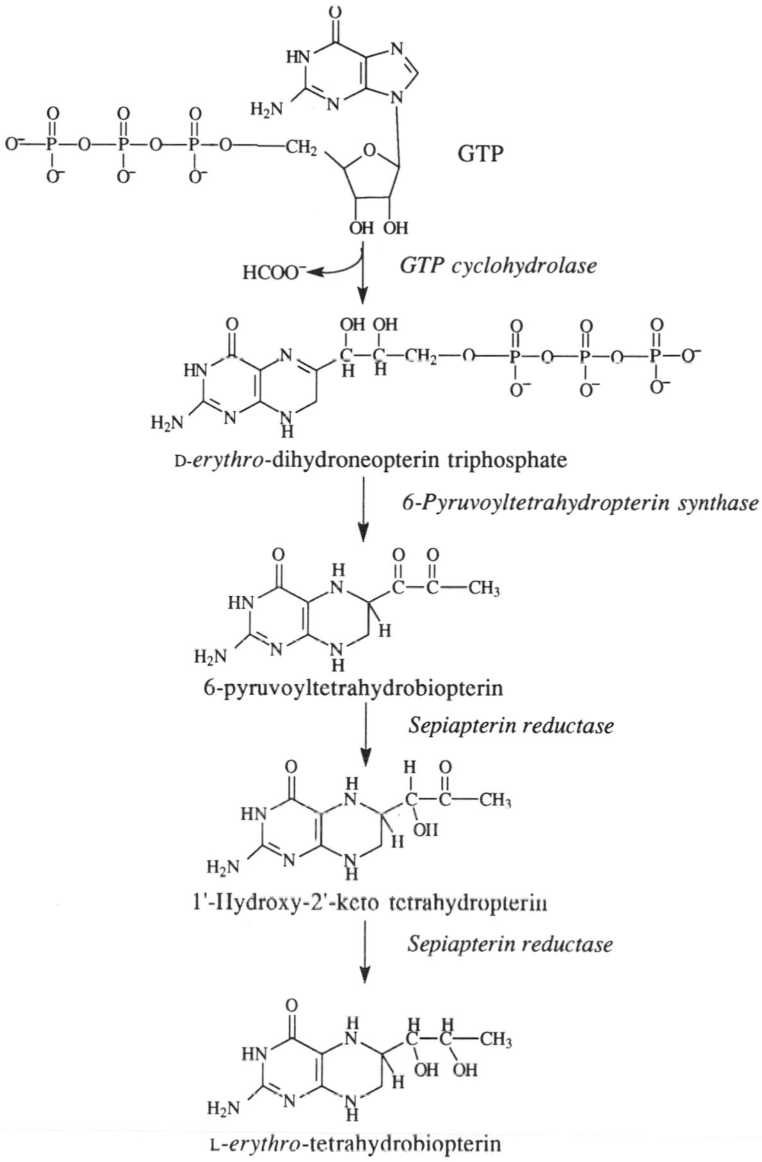

FIGURE A1-2. **Biosynthesis of tetrahydrobiopterin.**

d. Tetrahydrobiopterins are also involved as cofactors in biosynthesis of neurotransmitters such as norepinephrine and serotonin. The enzyme tyrosine hydroxylase, which converts tyrosine to 3,4-dihydroxyphenylalanine (DOPA), requires tetrahydrobiopterin, as does the enzyme tryptophan hydroxylase, which converts tryptophan to 5-hydroxytryptophan. It is not surprising, therefore, that a defect in biosynthesis of tetrahydrobiopterin would cause neurological problems.

An interesting question is why the presence of dihydrofolate reductase does not compensate for the defective dihydropteridine reductase, since dihydrofolate reductase can restore tetrahydrobiopterin from 7,8-dihydrobiopterin, and quinonoid dihydrobiopterin is an unstable compound that turns spontaneously into 7,8-dihydrobiopterin. Probably it is a quantitative question. The phenylalanine hydroxylase reaction and the other reactions that oxidize tetrahydrobiopterin generate quinonoid dihydrobiopterin at a certain rate. The latter spontaneously changes back to 7,8-dihydrobiopterin at a certain rate. Although dihydrofolate reductase can convert 7,8-dihydrobiopterin back to tetrahydrobiopterin,

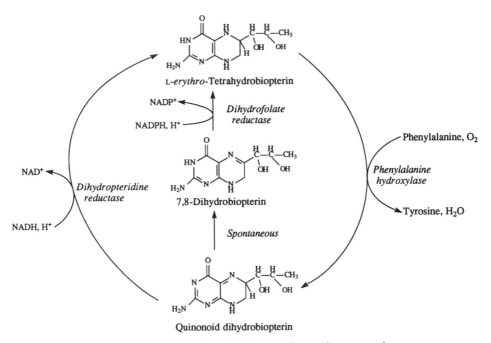

FIGURE A1-3. **Interrelationships among dihydropteridine reductase and dihydrofolate reductase.**

the rate at which this reaction proceeds is not sufficiently great to maintain an adequate supply of tetrahydrobiopterin. For this, it is necessary to have dihydropteridine reductase acting directly on the quinonoid dihydrobiopterin to convert it to tetrahydrobiopterin. The interrelationships among these enzymes are shown in Figure A1-3.

References

Brenneman, A. R., and Kaufman, S. The role of tetrahydropteridines in the enzymatic conversion of tyrosine to 3,4-dihydroxyphenylalanine. *Biochem. Biophys. Res. Commun.* 17: 177, 1964.

Burg, A. W., and Brown, G. M. The biosynthesis of folic acid. VIII. Purification and properties of the enzyme that catalyzes the production of formate from carbon atom 8 of guanosine triphosphate. *J. Biol. Chem.* 243: 2349, 1968.

Craine, J. E., Hall, E. S., and Kaufman, S. The isolation and characterization of dihydropteridine reductase from sheep liver. *J. Biol. Chem.* 247: 6082, 1972.

Friedman, P. A., Kappelman, A. H., and Kaufman, S. Partial purification and characterization of tryptophan hydroxylase from rabbit hindbrain. *J. Biol. Chem.* 247: 4165, 1972.

Kaufman, S. Metabolism of the phenylalanine hydroxylation cofactor. *J. Biol. Chem.* 242: 3934, 1967.

Kaufman, S., Holtzman, N. A., Milstien, S., Butler, I. J., and Krumholz, A. Phenylketonuria due to a deficiency of dihydropteridine reductase. *New Engl. J. Med.* 293: 785, 1975.

Scriver, C. R., Kaufman, S., and Woo, S. L. C. The hyperphenylalaninemias. C. R. Scriver, A. L. Beaudet, W. S. Sly, and D. Valle (Eds.). *The Metabolic Basis of Inherited Disease.* New York: McGraw-Hill, 1989, Vol. I, Chap. 15, p. 495.

Answer 2

a. Three enzymes are known to act on ornithine: (1) *ornithine transcarbamoylase*, (2) *ornithine decarboxylase*, and (3) *ornithine δ-aminotransferase*. Ornithine transcarboxylase is part of the urea cycle. A defect in this enzyme would block the urea cycle; although such a defect would greatly increase ornithine levels, ammonia levels would also greatly increase because the urea cycle would be impaired. The problem states that ammonia levels are normal, hence this is not a possibility. The enzyme ornithine decarboxylase converts ornithine to putrescine, a precursor of the polyamines, which are associated with DNA. The activity of this enzyme is

13

generally low except in rapidly dividing cells, such as bone marrow, embryonic, or tumor cells. Although a defect in this enzyme might elevate ornithine levels, the magnitude of the effect would probably be low. The most likely candidate for a defect in your patient, therefore, is *ornithine δ-aminotransferase* (Figure A2-1).

b. The level of Δ^1-pyrroline 5-carboxylate would probably be low, because ornithine inhibits the enzyme Δ^1-pyrroline 5-carboxylate synthase, which converts glutamate to Δ^1-pyrroline 5-carboxylate. High ornithine concentrations would inhibit the enzyme still more. The physiological significance in normal individuals of this action of ornithine is not clear.

c. The mutation in the patient is the conversion of a G to an A. It is not immediately clear that this is in the coding sequence, however.

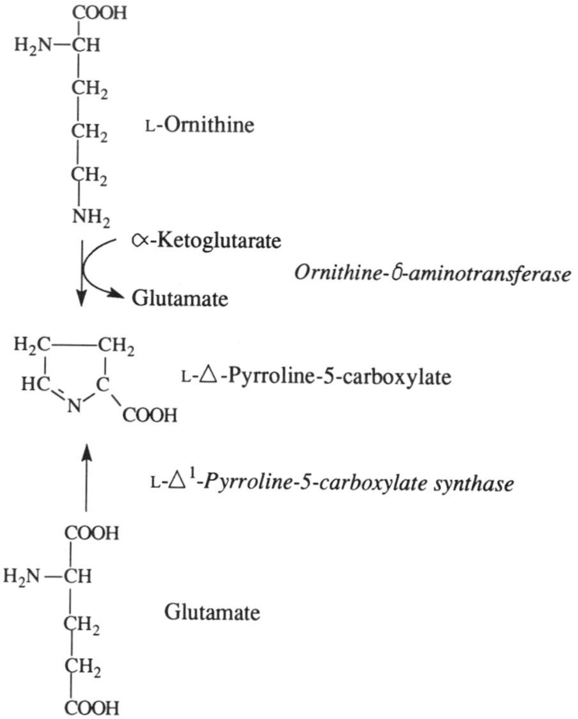

COOH
|
H_2N-CH
|
CH_2
|
CH_2 L-Ornithine
|
CH_2
|
NH_2
        α-Ketoglutarate

                    Ornithine-δ-aminotransferase

        Glutamate

H_2C——CH_2
| |
HC C L-Δ-Pyrroline-5-carboxylate
   \N/   \COOH

        L-Δ^1-Pyrroline-5-carboxylate synthase

COOH
|
H_2N-CH
|
CH_2 Glutamate
|
CH_2
|
COOH

FIGURE A2-1. **Biosynthesis of L-Δ^1-pyrroline-5-carboxylate.**

In the sequence from the normal person, the first methionine codon is ATG; in your patient, this is mutated to ATA, which codes for isoleucine. The ATG codon is likely to correspond to the N-terminal methionine, the site of initiation of translation. The mutation eliminates this methionine. Consequently, initiation would occur much later in the sequence and could be frameshifted as well. The probability of getting a functional enzyme is very low.

Your patient has GYRATE ATROPHY OF THE CHOROID AND RETINA.

References

Inana, G., Totsuka, S., Redmond, M., Dougherty, T., Nagle, J., Shiono, T., Ohura, T., Kominami, E., and Katunuma, N. Molecular cloning of human ornithine aminotransferase mRNA. *Proc. Natl. Acad. Sci. USA* 83: 1203, 1986.

Mitchell, G. A., Brody, L. C., Looney, J., Steel, G., Suchanek, M., Dowling, C., Der Kaloustian, V., Kaiser-Kupfer, M., and Valle, D. An initiator codon mutation in ornithine-δ-aminotransferase causing gyrate atrophy of the choroid and retina. *J. Clin. Invest.* 81: 630, 1988.

Ramesh, V., Shaffer, M. M., Allaire, J. M., Shih, V. E., and Gusella, J. F. Investigation of gyrate atrophy using a cDNA clone for human ornithine aminotransferase. *DNA* 5: 493, 1986.

Valle, D., and Simell, O. The hyperornithemias. C. R. Scriver, A. L. Beaudet, W. S. Sly, and D. Valle (Eds.). *The Metabolic Basis of Inherited Disease.* New York: McGraw-Hill, 1989, Vol. I, Chap. 19, p. 599.

Answer 3

a. Succinic semialdehyde is a metabolite of γ-aminobutyric acid (GABA). If its levels are elevated, one of the enzymes that metabolizes it must be defective. There are two such enzymes. One of these, succinic semialdehyde reductase, converts succinic semialdehyde to 4-hydroxybutyrate. This enzyme cannot be defective since we know that 4-hydroxybutyrate levels are high. The same argument would apply to the enzyme 4-hydroxybutyrate dehydrogenase, which converts 4-hydroxybutyrate to succinic semialdehyde; if this enzyme were overactive, succinic semialdehyde would indeed be high, but 4-hydroxybutyrate levels would be low, and this is not the case. Hence the defect must be

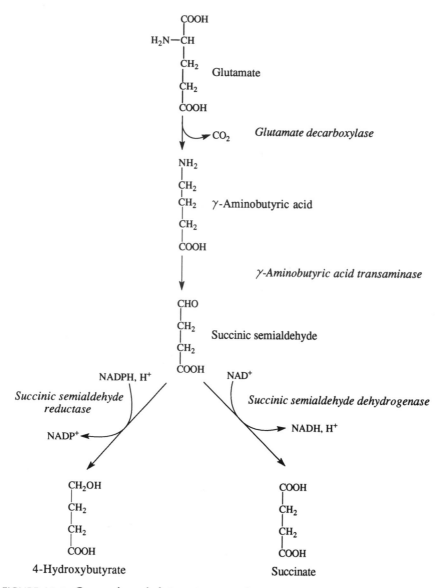

FIGURE A3-1. **Conversion of glutamate to succinate.**

in the other enzyme, *succinic semialdehyde dehydrogenase* (MW 191 kD), which converts succinic semialdehyde to succinate for entrance into the TCA cycle.

b. See Figure A3-1.

Your patient has 4-HYDROXYBUTYRIC ACIDURIA.

References

Chambliss, K. L., and Gibson, K. M. Succinic semialdehyde dehydrogenase from mammalian brain: subunit analysis using polyclonal antiserum. *Int. J. Biochem.* 24: 1493, 1992.

Cho, S.-W., Song, M.-S., Kim, G.-Y., Kang, W.-D., Choi, E. Y., and Choi, S. Y. Kinetics and mechanism of an NADPH-dependent succinic semialdehyde reductase from bovine brain. *Eur. J. Biochem.* 211: 757, 1993.

Jakobs, C., Jaeken, J., and Gibson, K. M. Inherited disorders of GABA metabolism. *J. Inherit. Metab. Dis.* 16: 704, 1993.

Scriver, C. R., and Perry, T. L. Disorders of ω-amino acids in free and peptide-linked forms. C. R. Scriver, A. L. Beaudet, W. S. Sly, and D. Valle (Eds.). *The Metabolic Basis of Inherited Disease.* New York: McGraw-Hill, 1989, Vol. I, Chap. 26, p. 755.

Tunnicliff, G. Significance of γ-hydroxybutyric acid in the brain. *Gen. Pharmacol.* 23: 1027, 1992.

Answer 4

a. Your patient's serum levels of tryptophan are lower than normal. This would imply one of the following: (1) tryptophan is being poorly absorbed; (2) tryptophan is being metabolized at a much higher rate than normal (increased catabolism); or (3) tryptophan is being excreted at higher-than-normal rates (i.e., there could be a defect in the reabsorption in the kidney). The third possibility can be eliminated because it would imply high concentrations of tryptophan in the urine, and what you actually find is that these are low. The second possibility is more complicated. None of the normal catabolites of tryptophan, generated by mammalian enzymes, are blue. However, bacteria can metabolize tryptophan into indigo blue. Thus the second possibility is unlikely because increased catabolism caused by excess activity of one of our enzymes would not account for the blue color. This leaves the first possibility. If tryptophan is not absorbed well by the intestine, it will remain in the intestine and become catabolized by the resident bacteria. One of the end products of tryptophan's renal catabolism is indigo blue. It seems that the most likely solution to the problem is a defect in the protein which transports tryptophan into the intestine. The indigo blue that your patient's bacteria produce is absorbed by the intestine and excreted in the urine, giving it a blue color.

b. See Figure A4-1.

Your patient has BLUE DIAPER SYNDROME.

References

Budavari, S. *The Merck Index: An Encyclopedia of Chemicals, Drugs, and Biologicals,* 11th Ed. Rahway, NJ: Merck & Co., Inc., 1989, p. 784.

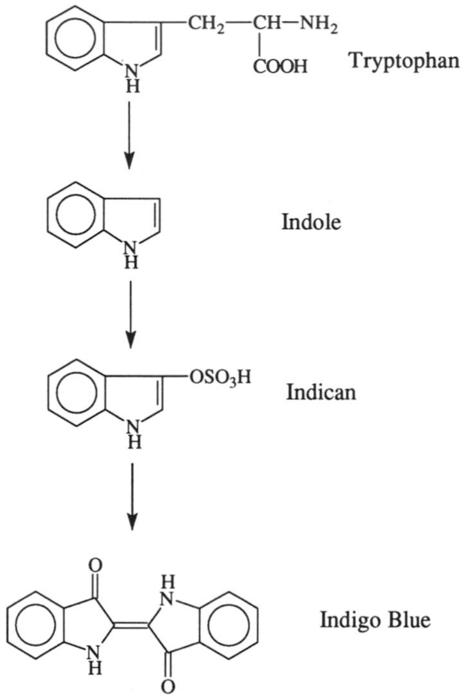

FIGURE A4-1. **Conversion of tryptophan to indigo blue in the gut.**

Drummond, K. N., Michael, A. F., Ulstrom, R. A., and Good, R. A. The blue diaper syndrome: familial hypercalcemia with nephrocalcinosis and indicanuria. *Am. J. Med.* 37: 928, 1964.

Levy, H. L. Hartnup disorder. C. R. Scriver, A. L. Beaudet, W. S. Sly, and D. Valle (Eds.). *The Metabolic Basis of Inherited Disease.* New York: McGraw-Hill, 1989, Vol. II, Chap. 101, p. 2515.

Answer 5

a. Your patient has excessive levels in his urine and feces of a variety of uncharged amino acids. Blood levels, however, are low. This is not a generalized disorder of protein metabolism, since otherwise all amino acids would be affected. In principle, there are four possibilities to consider.

1. Excessive catabolism of these amino acids could account for their low blood levels, but the high levels in the feces and urine rule this out; it is also hard to imagine a single defect in catabolism that would affect these disparate amino acids whose metabolic fates are very different.

2. Poor renal reabsorption of these amino acids would account for the high urinary and low blood levels but not explain the high fecal levels.

3. Poor intestinal absorption would explain the high fecal and low blood levels but not the high urinary levels.

4. A combination of the second and third possibilities would do the trick; in other words, impaired absorption in the intestine and reabsorption in the kidney would explain the low levels in blood and high levels in feces and urine. However, the fourth possibility would imply that a single protein, such as a transport protein, would mediate both intestinal absorption and renal reabsorption. This is indeed correct. There is a transporter of neutral amino acids that operates in both the intestine and the kidney. It is this transporter that is defective in your patient.

b. Nicotinamide is low in your patient's blood. Although nicotinamide is a vitamin present in a normal diet, a certain amount of nicotinamide is made from tryptophan by the pathway shown in Figures A5-1

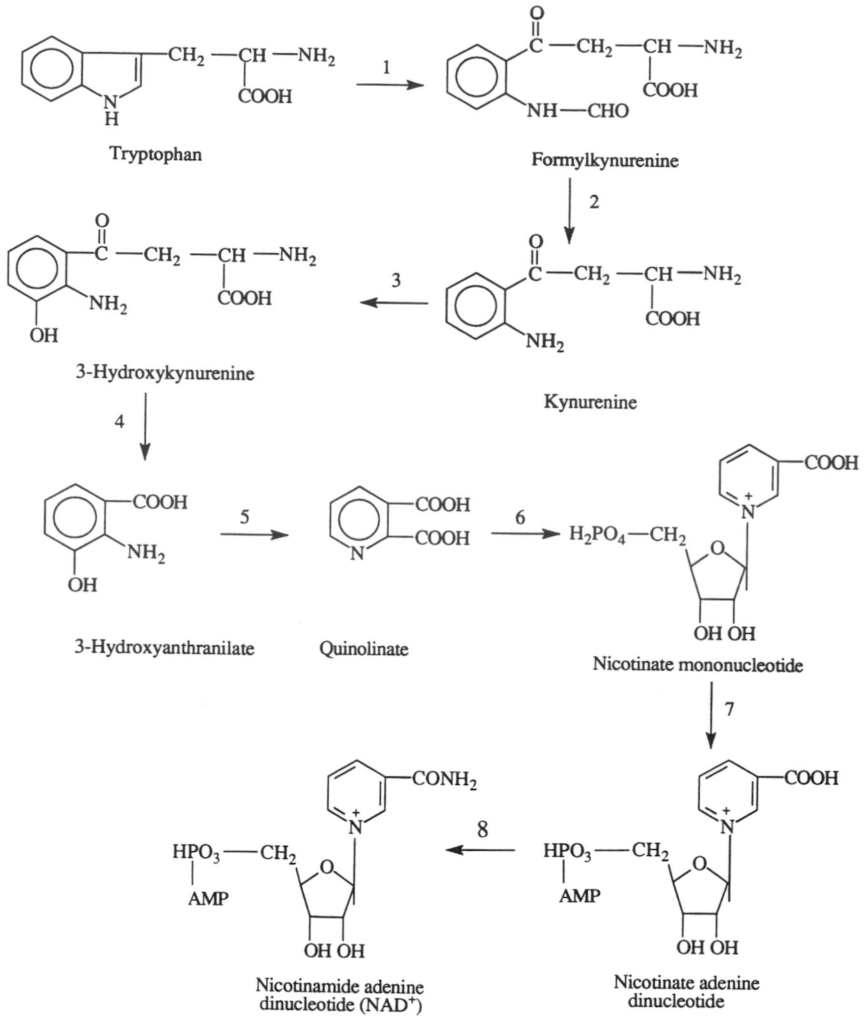

FIGURE A5-1. **Biosynthesis of NAD$^+$. Enzymes are numbered as follows: 1, tryptophan oxygenase; 2, kynurenine formamidase; 3, kynurenine hydroxylase; 4, kynureninase; 5, 3-hydroxyanthranilate oxidase; 6, quinolinate phosphoribosyl transferase; 7, NAD-pyrophosphorylase; 8, NAD synthetase.**

and A5-2. Since your patient has trouble absorbing tryptophan, the concentration of tryptophan in his cells is too low to do more than support protein synthesis; hence there is not enough to make nicotinamide adenine nucleotide (NAD$^+$) or its derivative NADP$^+$, which are essential

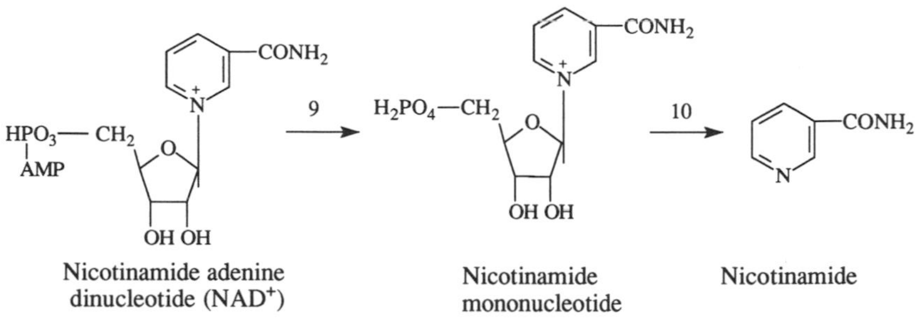

FIGURE A5-2. **Biosynthesis of nicotinamide. Enzymes are numbered as follows: 9, NAD-pyrophosphorylase; 10, nicotinamide phosphoribosyl transferase.**

coenzymes. If the nicotinamide levels are low, NAD^+ levels must be low as well.

Your patient has HARTNUP DISORDER.

References

Cory, J. G. Purine and pyrimidine nucleotide metabolism. T. M. Devlin (Ed.). *Textbook of Biochemistry with Clinical Correlations.* New York: Wiley-Liss, 1992, Chap. 13, p. 529.

Levy, H. L. Hartnup disorder. C. R. Scriver, A. L. Beaudet, W. S. Sly, and D. Valle (Eds.). *The Metabolic Basis of Inherited Disease.* New York: McGraw-Hill, 1989, Vol. II, Chap. 101, p. 2515.

Answer 6

a. If glycine, proline, and hydroxyproline are elevated in the urine, there is clearly not a problem in uptake in the intestine. If their levels in the blood are within normal limits, there is not a problem with metabolism. Since these three amino acids occur in large amounts in collagen, one might imagine that an increase in degradation of collagen would account for the elevated excretion of these amino acids, but the normal blood levels preclude this interpretation. The solution must be a problem in reabsorbing them in the kidney. It turns out that there is a transport protein in the kidney specific for these three amino acids. Thus the defective protein is the *renal carrier for imino acids and glycine.*

b. If these two patients differ in that one has lower levels of these amino acids in the urine than does the other patient, and we cannot invoke another protein, the two patients must differ in the nature of the defect in their transport protein. A difference in affinity would explain the observations. The second patient's carrier protein would have higher affinity for these amino acids than does the carrier protein of the first patient.

c. These three amino acids are nonessential in our diets. Glycine and proline can be made in the body from precursors. Hydroxyproline is produced in molecules such as collagen by posttranslational modification or proline residues. Your patient will compensate for the increased excretion of proline and glycine by an increase in their biosynthesis. Hence the condition is symptom-free. The only potential problem might be during starvation. Your patient might be more susceptible since he will lose more amino acids than would a normal person.

Your patients have FAMILIAL RENAL IMINOGLYCINURIA.

Reference

Scriver, C. R. Familial renal iminoglycinuria. C. R. Scriver, A. L. Beaudet, W. S. Sly, and D. Valle (Eds.). *The Metabolic Basis of Inherited Disease.* New York: McGraw-Hill, 1989, Vol. II, Chap. 102, p. 2529.

Answer 7

a. The metabolic defect in your patient suggests that he lacks the enzyme that cleaves glycylproline into glycine and proline. This enzyme, a dipeptidase, is called *prolidase*. Prolidase catalyzes the reaction shown in Figure A7-1.

b. Your patient has high levels of hydroxyproline in his fibroblasts. Since collagen is by far the major protein that contains hydroxyproline, this is a clue that points to collagen as a problem. Collagen has an amino acid sequence in which glycine is at every third position and proline content is very high. You would expect that in normal turnover of

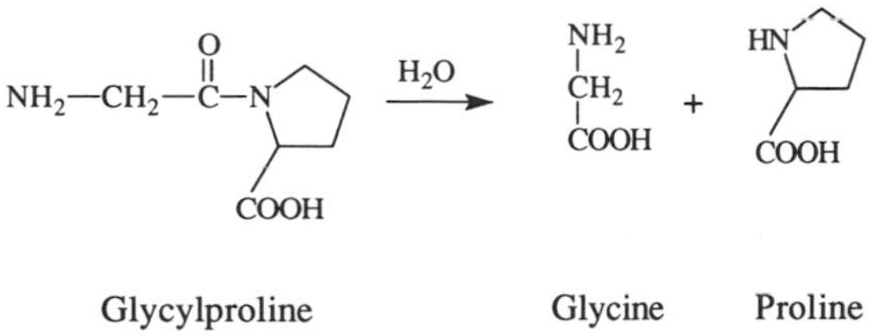

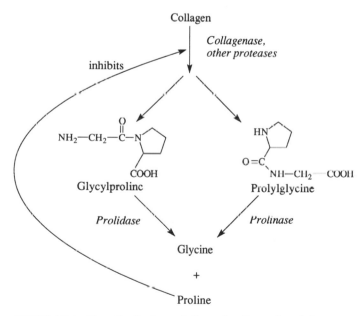

NH₂—CH₂—C—N ... (O) ... H₂O → NH₂ CH₂ COOH + HN COOH

COOH

Glycylproline   Glycine   Proline

FIGURE A7-1. **Cleavage of glycylproline by prolidase.**

collagen, you would get as catabolic intermediates, dipeptides with proline as either the C-terminal or N-terminal residue. Dipeptides with C-
terminal proline, such as glycylproline, are broken down by the enzyme
prolidase, as already mentioned. Dipeptides with N-terminal proline are
digested by the enzyme *prolinase*, in which to date no defect has been
reported. The high levels of dipeptides with C-terminal proline in your
patient's urine suggests a problem with collagen breakdown and also point
to prolidase, rather than prolinase, as the defective enzyme.

Collagen

*Collagenase,
other proteases*

inhibits

NH₂—CH₂—C—N (O) ... HN ... O=C, NH—CH₂—COOH

COOH
Glycylproline   Prolylglycine

Prolidase   *Prolinase*

Glycine

+

Proline

FIGURE A7-2. **Hypothetical regulation of collagen breakdown.**

The high levels of hydroxyproline suggest that collagen degradation is increased. Perhaps collagen degradation is controlled by the level of proline, and in the absence of prolidase, the concentration of free proline is lower and hence more collagen degradation occurs. Abnormal collagen metabolism could cause skin problems. One could postulate a scheme for regulating collagen breakdown (Figure A7-2).

References

Butterworth, J., and Priestman, D. A. Presence in human cells and tissues of two prolidases and their alteration in prolidase deficiency. *J. Inherit. Metab. Dis.* 8: 193, 1985.

Endo, F., Tanoue, A., Hata, A., Kitano, A., and Matsuda, I. Deduced amino acid sequence of human prolidase and molecular analyses of prolidase deficiency. *J. Inherit. Metab. Dis.* 12: 351, 1989.

Myara, I., Charpentier, C., and Lemonnier, A. Minireview: prolidase and prolidase deficiency. *Life Sci.* 34: 1985, 1984.

Phang, J. M., and Scriver, C. R. Disorders of proline and hydroxyproline metabolism. C. R. Scriver, A. L. Beaudet, W. S. Sly, and D. Valle (Eds.). *The Metabolic Basis of Inherited Disease.* New York: McGraw-Hill, 1989, Vol. I, Chap. 18, p. 577.

Answer 8

a. Your patient's melanocytes cannot transform added tyrosine into melanin, but a cell-free extract prepared from those melanocytes carries out this reaction perfectly well. This implies that the defective protein must be involved with uptake of tyrosine into the melanocytes. This is consistent with the observation that the defective protein has 12 hydrophobic domains, suggesting that it is a membrane protein. Lacking the protein, tyrosine does not enter the melanocytes and is unable to be converted into melanin. Lack of melanin causes albinism and the other symptoms.

b. Your other patient has the exact same symptoms but is missing part of chromosome 15. Unless this is just a coincidence, this implies that the gene for the tyrosine transport protein is probably located on the missing part of chromosome 15.

Your patient has **TYPE II OCULOCUTANEOUS ALBINISM.**

Reference

Witkop, C. J., Quevedo, W. C., Fitzpatrick, T. B., and King, R. A. Albinism. C. R. Scriver, A. L. Beaudet, W. S. Sly, and D. Valle (Eds.). *The Metabolic Basis of Inherited Disease.* New York: McGraw-Hill, 1989, Vol. II, Chap. 119, p. 2905.

CHAPTER 2

Nucleotides

Problem 9

Your patient has colic, blood in his urine, and kidney stones. The stones are made of 2,8-dihydroxyadenine. He has high urinary levels of adenine, 8-hydroxyadenine, and 2,8-dihydroxyadenine. He lives in a vegetarian commune whose members consume in their diet large quantities of lentils and other grains and vegetables rich in adenine. You find that putting your patient on a low-purine diet greatly helps his symptoms.

a. Name the defective enzyme.

b. Describe the reaction catalyzed by this enzyme.

Problem 10

Your patient is a 44-year-old man with a relatively mild problem. Every time he does exercise, he feels excessively tired and often has muscle cramps. You do a muscle biopsy. You prepare a cell-free extract from the biopsied tissue and add adenosine monophosphate (AMP) labeled with ^{15}N. You measure the production of labeled ammonia and compare the results with those obtained from a normal person. You find that the production of ammonia in the cell extract prepared from your patient is about 1% as great as that from a cell extract of a normal person.

    a. Name the defective enzyme and show the reaction that it catalyzes.

    b. Write out the cycle in which this enzyme is involved.

Problem 11

Your patient is a 27-year-old woman with breast cancer. You are treating her with 5-fluorouracil (5-FU). She has a very severe neurological reaction to 5-FU. Her urinary levels of uracil and thymine are very high.

    a. Name the defective enzyme and show the reaction that it catalyzes.

    b. Show the pathways in which this enzyme plays a part.

    c. Why do you think the 5-FU was so toxic for your patient?

Problem 12

Your patient is a 39-year-old man with bladder stones. Analysis of the stones shows that they are made of uric acid (Figure P12-1). Your patient's urine has a high concentration of uric acid, but the concentration in his blood is very low. He has a high concentration of calcium in his urine. Other substances in the urine and blood are present at normal concentrations.

a. What is the deficiency in your patient?

b. Is your patient likely to get gout? Why or why not?

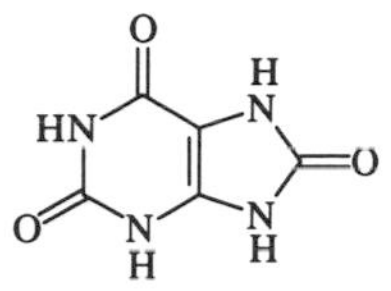

Uric acid

FIGURE P12-1. **Structure of uric acid.**

Answer 9

a. Your patient clearly has trouble disposing of excess adenine, suggesting that the defective enzyme is involved in the metabolism of adenine. Two enzymes act on adenine. One, *adenine phosphoribosyl transferase,* converts adenine to adenylic acid which is then metabolized to uric acid for excretion. The other, *xanthine oxidase,* converts adenine to 8-hydroxyadenine and 2,8-dihydroxyadenine. The second enzyme cannot be the defective one, since production of 8-hydroxyadenine and 2,8-dihydroxyadenine is not impaired but, in fact, enhanced. Logically, therefore, the defective enzyme must be *adenine phosphoribosyl transferase.* A defect in this enzyme would channel excess adenine toward the xanthine oxidase pathway, resulting in an excess of 8-hydroxyadenine and 2,8-dihydroxyadenine. Under normal circumstances, xanthine oxidase does not use adenine as a substrate because adenine concentrations are maintained at a low level by the action of adenine phosphoribosyl transferase.

b. See Figure A9-1.

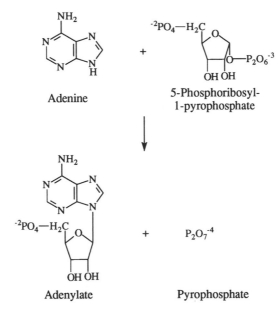

FIGURE A9-1. **Reaction catalyzed by adenine phosphoribosyl transferase.**

Reference

Simmonds, H. A., Sahota, A. S., and Van Acker, K. J. Adenine phosphoribosyltransfer-
ase deficiency and 2,8-dihydroxyadenine lithiasis. C. R. Scriver, A. L. Beaudet,
W. S. Sly, and D. Valle (Eds.). *The Metabolic Basis of Inherited Disease.* New York:
McGraw-Hill, 1989, Vol. I, Chap. 39, p. 1029.

Answer 10

a. The defective enzyme is clearly the one that removes ammonia
from AMP. This enzyme is AMP deaminase. However, this enzyme exists
in four isozymes. One of these isozymes appears to be restricted to skeletal
muscle. Since your patient's symptoms also appear to be only muscular,
it is likely that only the skeletal muscle isozyme is defective. This isozyme
is called *myoadenylate deaminase.* The reaction that this enzyme catalyzes
is shown in Figure A10-1.

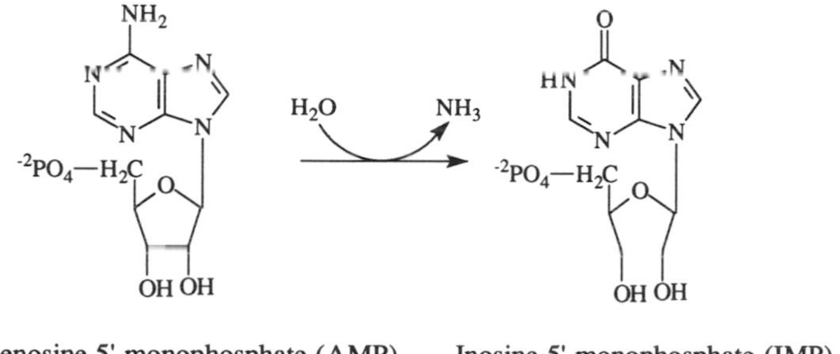

Adenosine 5'-monophosphate (AMP)   Inosine 5'-monophosphate (IMP)

FIGURE A10-1. **Myoadenylate deaminase reaction.**

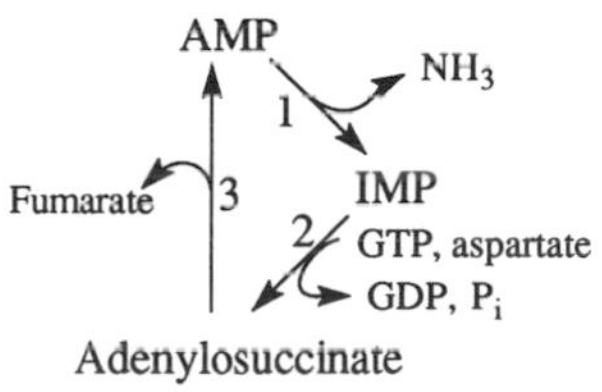

FIGURE A10-2. **Myoadenylate deaminase is part of a cycle. The enzymes are
as follows: 1, myoadenylate deaminase; 2, adenylosuccinate synthetase;
3, adenylosuccinate lyase.**

b. The reaction catalyzed by myoadenylate deaminase is part of a purine nucleotide cycle (Figure A10-2).

References

Sabina, R. L., Swain, J. L., and Holmes, E. W. Myoadenylate deaminase deficiency. C. R. Scriver, A. L. Beaudet, W. S. Sly, and D. Valle (Eds.). *The Metabolic Basis of Inherited Disease*. New York: McGraw-Hill, 1989, Vol. I, Chap. 41, p. 1077.

Smith, E. L., Hill, R. L., Lehman, I. R., Lefkowitz, R. J., Handler, P., and White, A. *Principles of Biochemistry: Mammalian Biochemistry*. New York: McGraw-Hill, 1983.

Answer 11

a. Elevated levels of uracil and thymine suggest a defect in their catabolism. Three enzymes are involved here: *dihydropyrimidine dehydrogenase, hydropyrimidine hydrase,* and *ureidopropionase.* Uracil and thymine are converted, respectively, to dihydrouracil and dihydrothymine by dihydropyrimidine dehydrogenase. Dihydrouracil is converted to ureidopropionic acid by hydropyrimidine hydrase and then to β-alanine by ureidopropionase. Entirely analogously, the same two enzymes metabolize dihydrothymine to β-ureidoisobutyric acid and then to β-aminoisobutyric acid. The fact that only uracil and thymine are present in excess suggests that the defective enzyme is the one that acts directly on uracil and thymine, namely *dihydropyrimidine dehydrogenase.* The reactions catalyzed by this enzyme are shown in Figure A11-1.

b. See Figure A11-1.

c. 5-FU (Figure A11-2) is metabolized by dihydropyrimidine dehydrogenase. If the enzyme is defective, levels of 5-FU will remain high and cause toxicity. The levels of 5-FU will remain higher than the normal therapeutic dose.

References

Bakkeren, J. A. J. M., De Abreu, R. A., Sengers, R. C. A., Gabreëls, F. J. M., Maas, J. M., and Renier, W. O. Elevated urine, blood and cerebrospinal fluid levels of uracil and thymine in a child with dihydrothymine dehydrogenase deficiency. *Clin. Chim. Acta* 140: 247, 1984.

Fritzson, P. Properties and assay of dihydrouracil dehydrogenase of rat liver. *J. Biol. Chem.* 235: 719, 1960.

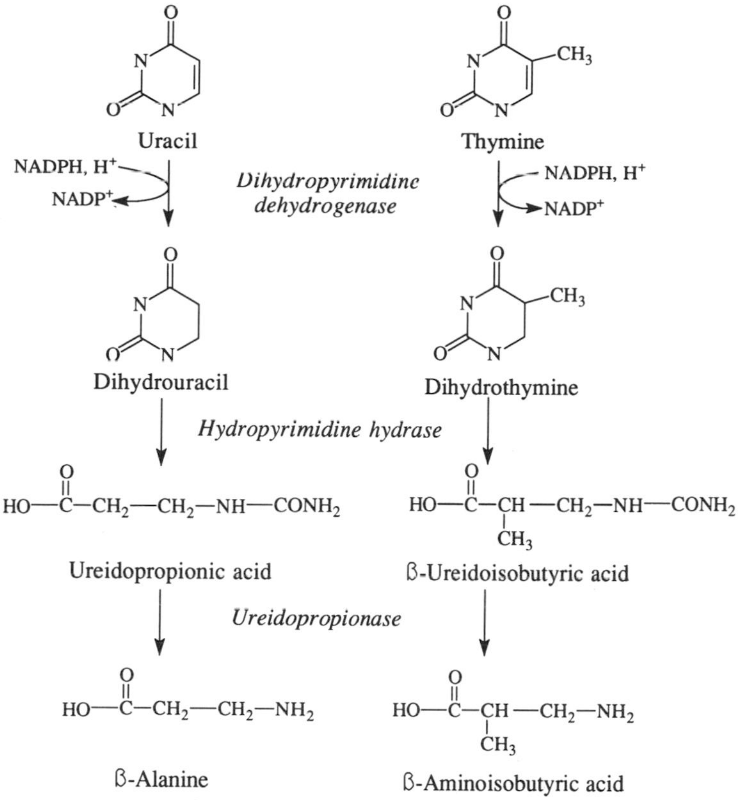

FIGURE A11-1. **Catabolism of uracil and thymine.**

Grisolia, S., and Cardoso, S. S. The purification and properties of hydropyrimidine dehydrogenase. *Biochim. Biophys. Acta* 25: 430, 1957.

Shiotani, T., and Weber, G. Purification and properties of dihydrothymine dehydrogenase from rat liver. *J. Biol. Chem.* 256: 219, 1981.

Suttle, D. P., Becroft, D. M. O., and Webster, D. R. Hereditary orotic aciduria and other disorders of pyrimidine metabolism. C. R. Scriver, A. L. Beaudet, W. S. Sly, and D. Valle (Eds.). *The Metabolic Basis of Inherited Disease.* New York: McGraw-Hill, 1989, Vol. I, Chap. 43, p. 1095.

Answer 12

a. If uric acid levels are high in the urine and low in the blood, this implies that there is a problem with the transport of uric acid in the

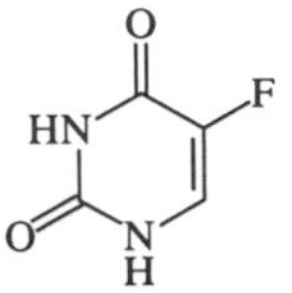

FIGURE A11-2. **Structure of 5-fluorouracil.**

kidney. This could be part of a general problem with transport in the kidney, but we are told specifically that other substances in the urine and blood are present at normal concentrations. The movement of urate in the kidney is complex. First, some urate passes from the blood into the glomerulus. Then it is reabsorbed in the early proximal tubule. Following this, urate is secreted into the later proximal tubule. Then urate is reabsorbed again still later in the proximal tubule, shortly before entering the renal medulla. In principle, any one of these four processes could be defective in such a way as to increase the amount of urate in the urine and decrease it in the blood. A defect in glomerular filtration to permit higher excretion of urate is unlikely, because it is difficult to imagine this being specific for urate. Hence we either have decreased reabsorption or increased secretion. So far, this defect has never been traced to increased secretion. Thus the defect is in the *renal urate uptake system*. Excessive calcium in the urine also characterizes many of the people who have this disease; however, the reason for this association is not known.

b. Your patient is not likely to get gout, because the urate level in his blood is always low. Gout is caused by excess of urate, which is deposited as crystals in the joints.

Your patient has HEREDITARY RENAL HYPOURICEMIA.

Reference

Sperling, O. Hereditary renal hypouricemia. C. R. Scriver, A. L. Beaudet, W. S. Sly, and D. Valle (Eds.). *The Metabolic Basis of Inherited Disease.* New York: McGraw-Hill, 1989, Vol. II, Chap. 106, p. 2605.

CHAPTER 3

Carbohydrate Metabolism

Problem 13

Your patient is a 23-year-old soldier who has generally been asymptomatic. Another doctor examined him before he enlisted and observed a high level of glucose in his urine. At first, he was not allowed to enlist because it was suspected that he was a diabetic. However, it was determined that the insulin level in his blood was normal. When he took a glucose tolerance test, his blood glucose rose quickly and then fell, exactly as in any normal (nondiabetic) person. While fighting in the desert he collapsed from dehydration and was sent home for R&R. You did some further examinations on him. You repeated the results observed by the earlier doctor and observed that the sugar which was elevated in his urine was D-glucose and that no other sugar was elevated. Glucose absorption from his gut appeared to be normal.

a. In which protein is your patient deficient, and what does that protein do?

b. Why is he more susceptible to dehydration and starvation?

Problem 14

Your patient is a 20-year-old man who was normal at birth but soon exhibited delay in development of intellectual and motor skills. He has high levels of sialic acid in his urine and his blood. You culture his fibroblasts and find that the intracellular level of sialic acid is high. Particularly high concentrations are present in the lysosomes. You do an experiment in which you add a radioactive sialic acid derivative to his lysosomes and find that the rate at which the sialic acid leaves the lysosomes is very low compared to that which you would expect to find for a normal person. You measure the intracellular activities of N-acetylneuraminate lyase, sialidase, CMP-N-acylneuraminate phosphodiesterase, and acylneuraminate cytidylyl transferase and find that they are all normal.

a. What is the likely defect in your patient?

b. What is the origin of the intralysosomal sialic acid?

c. Write out the pathway by which N-acetylneuraminic acid is metabolized.

Problem 15

Your patient is a Greenland Eskimo who is living in the continental United States for the first time in her life. She developed a liking for pizza and would eat a tomato-and-cheese pizza every other day with no problems. One day, she ate a very fancy pizza containing pepperoni, sausage, olives, green peppers, mushrooms, tomatoes, and cheese. She soon developed diarrhea and vomiting. You recovered some of her intestinal fluid and found a very high concentration of trehalose in it.

    a. Name the defective enzyme and state what it does.

    b. Describe the structure of trehalose.

    c. What common food is the only one that contains significant quantities of trehalose?

Problem 16

Your patient is a 5-year-old boy with an enlarged liver and spleen, numerous skeletal deformities, and hearing loss. He has frequent diarrhea, bronchitis, and earaches. He has high levels of dermatan sulfate and heparan sulfate in his urine. You draw some blood and do an assay in which you add dermatan sulfate labeled with radioactive [^{35}S]sulfate at the number 2 position of the terminal L-iduronic acid residue. You find that release of label is 3% of that of a normal person.

    a. Name the defective enzyme.

    b. Write out the pathway in which this enzyme occurs (e.g., write down the pathway of degradation of dermatan sulfate).

Problem 17

Your patient is a 10-year-old girl who was normal until age 5, when she learned how to read and write. She then underwent severe mental degeneration. She is no longer able to read or write and has difficulty constructing sentences. She has frequent temper tantrums and appears to have the emotional maturity of a 3-year-old. Her physical symptoms are minimal except for some hearing loss. She has high levels of heparan sulfate in her urine. You draw some blood and do an assay in which you add heparan sulfate labeled with radioactive sulfate on the nitrogen of the terminal glucosamine residue and you find that release of labeled sulfate is only 1% of that observed with blood of a normal person.

    a. Name the defective enzyme.

    b. Write out the pathway in which this enzyme occurs.

Problem 18

Your patient has severe skeletal deformities. He also has cloudy corneas. You draw some blood and do an assay in which you add keratan sulfate labeled with radioactive sulfate at carbon 6 in the terminal galactose residue. You measure release of radioactive sulfate and find that it is 12% of that which you would find with a normal person.

a. Name the defective enzyme.

b. Write out the pathway in which this enzyme occurs.

Answer 13

a. Your patient does not have diabetes because he has no trouble clearing glucose from his blood. The fact that the elevation of sugar is increased in his urine implies that the problem may lie in his kidney. Occasionally, a malformed kidney could have problems with reabsorption, but this is almost certainly not the problem with your patient because the defect seems to involve only D-glucose and no other sugar. Since the problem appears to be a defect in the renal reabsorption of glucose, the defect is likely to be in a *renal glucose transporter*. If such a protein is defective, glucose concentrations in the urine will be high.

Our bodies contain several glucose transport proteins. Among these are the facilitative glucose transporters GLUT1, GLUT2, GLUT3, GLUT4, and GLUT5, which facilitate glucose transport along its concentration gradient. In addition there are the Na^+/glucose cotransporters which can pump glucose against a concentration gradient in a process powered by the sodium concentration gradient; this latter category includes one well categorized protein called SGLT1 and others less well-known. Of these proteins, the kidney contains GLUT2, SGLT1, and another, less well-characterized Na^+/glucose cotransporter. SGLT1 is unlikely to be the candidate because it has similar affinities for glucose and galactose and your patient's abnormality in transport appears to involve only glucose. Also, SGLT1 plays a major role in glucose absorption in the intestine which appears to be normal in your patient. GLUT2 is also an unlikely candidate because it is located in the liver, intestine and the β-cell of the pancreas as well as the kidney. Hence, a defect in GLUT2 may have many more serious effects than your patient manifests. The likely defect is in the other Na^+/glucose cotransporter since that one is known to have a very high specificity for glucose.

b. Your patient loses glucose more quickly because of the failure to reabsorb. He gets dehydrated because water is reabsorbed with glucose. In a stressful situation, he will lose water a little faster than would a normal person.

Your patient has RENAL GLYCOSURIA.

Reference

Desjeux, J.-F. Congenital selective Na$^+$, D-glucose cotransport defects leading to renal glycosuria and congenital selective intestinal malabsorption of glucose and galactose. C. R. Scriver, A. L. Beaudet, W. S. Sly, and D. Valle (Eds.). *The Metabolic Basis of Inherited Disease.* New York: McGraw-Hill, 1989, Vol. II, Chap. 98, p. 2463.

Elsas, L. J., and Longo, N. "Glucose transporters." *Annu. Rev. Med.* 43: 377, 1992.

Answer 14

a. The excessive concentrations of sialic acid in the blood and urine suggest that there is a problem in the metabolism of sialic acid, that either too much is made or too little is broken down. If too much sialic acid is released from glycoproteins as a result of the action of unusually active sialidase, this could account for the high sialic acid. However, sialidase activity is normal. If there was a defect in metabolizing sialic acid, one of the following enzymes would have to be defective and operating at lower levels: acylneuraminate cytidylyl transferase, which transfers sialic acid onto CMP, or N-acetylneuraminate lyase, which breaks down sialic acid into N-acetylmannosamine and pyruvate; these enzymes are normal, however. Finally, if there was an overactive CMP-N-acylneuraminate phosphodiesterase, we would have excess sialic acid, since this enzyme releases sialic acid from CMP. Yet this enzyme, too, is normal. It thus seems that sialic acid metabolism is normal. The experiment involving adding the radioactive sialic acid derivative to a preparation of lysosomes points us in another direction and suggests that the lysosomes accumulate excessive sialic acid and shows that sialic acid leaves the lysosome much more slowly than normal. This, in turn, implies that the defect is in the *lysosomal membrane-free sialic carrier.* This conclusion is corroborated by the observation that other enzymes involved in the metabolism of sialic acid are present at normal activities.

b. One of the jobs of the lysosome is to break down macromolecules such as glycoproteins. These often contain carbohydrate moieties such as sialic acid. Thus the origin of the sialic acid is in glycoconjugates.

c. See Figure A14-1.

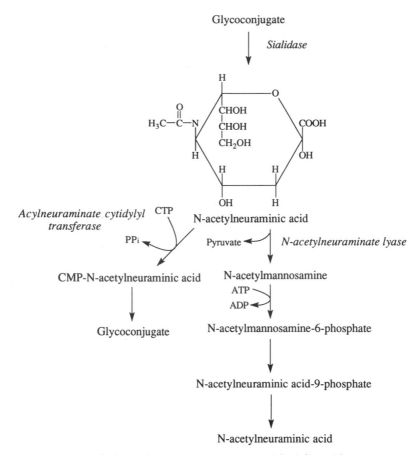

FIGURE A14-1. **Metabolism of *N*-acetylneuraminic acid (sialic acid).**

Your patient has SALLA DISEASE.

References

Gahl W. A., Renlund, M., and Thoene, J. G. Lysosomal transport disorders: cystinosis and sialic acid storate disorders. C. R. Scriver, A. L. Beaudet, W. S. Sly, and D. Valle (Eds.). *The Metabolic Basis of Inherited Disease.* New York: McGraw-Hill, 1989, Vol. II, Chap. 107, p. 2619.

Schwartz, N. B. Carbophydrate metabolism II: special pathways. T. M. Devlin (Ed.). *Textbook of Biochemistry with Clinical Correlations.* New York: Wiley-Liss, 1992, Chap. 8, p. 359.

Answer 15

a. Trehalose is a disaccharide. The brush border of the cells of the small intestine contains a variety of enzymes, such as sucrase, maltase, lactase, and trehalase; each of these enzymes can cleave disaccharides. Trehalase cleaves trehalose into two glucoses.

b. Trehalose has the structure α-D-glycopyranosyl-α-D-glucopyranoside (Figure A15-1).

c. Trehalose is a rare disaccharide. It is found normally only in mushrooms and in insects. It is particularly concentrated in young mushrooms where it accounts for 1.4% of their mass. The mushrooms on the pizza would have caused your patient's problem. Since the trehalose is undigested in your patient's intestine, it is metabolized anaerobically by the intestinal flora, thereby causing diarrhea and other symptoms. In general, when sugars are poorly absorbed in the gut, the intestinal flora metabolize them to give gases such as CO_2 and H_2 and small organic acids such as acetic, propionic, butyric and lactic acids. These compounds together with the undigested trehalose, could create an osmotic gradient which would cause water to flow from the plasma into the gut. The end result is abdominal pain and diarrhea.

Trehalase deficiency is found in 10 to 15% of Greenland Eskimos. Presumably, since their normal diet is heavy in fish and fish-eating mammals, they do not consume either mushrooms or insects. Hence there is no selective advantage for an Eskimo to have trehalase.

References

Gudmund-Hoyer, E., Fenger, H. J., Skovbjerg, H., Kern-Hansen, P., and Rorbaek Madsen, P. "Trehalase deficiency in Greenland." *Scand. J. Gastroenterol.* 23: 775, 1988.

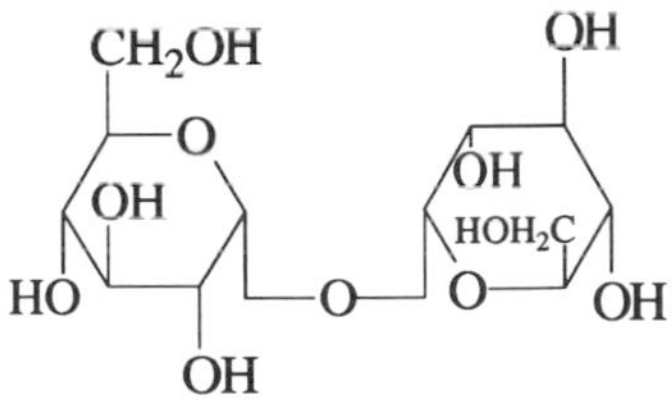

FIGURE A15-1. **Structure of trehalose.**

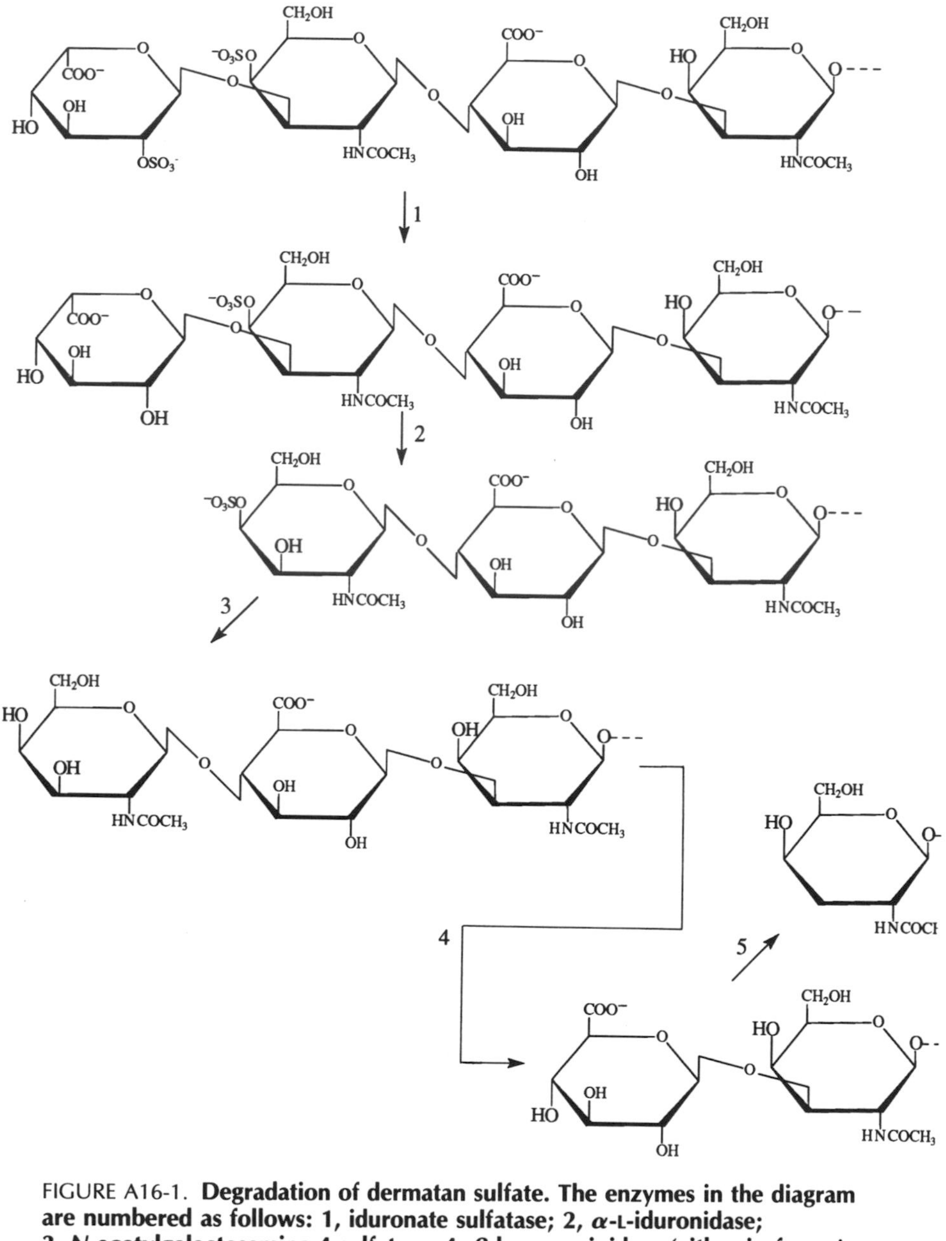

FIGURE A16-1. **Degradation of dermatan sulfate. The enzymes in the diagram are numbered as follows: 1, iduronate sulfatase; 2, α-L-iduronidase; 3, N-acetylgalactosamine 4-sulfatase; 4, β-hexosaminidase (either isoform A or isoform B); 5, β-glucuronidase.**

Harries, J. T. "Disorders of carbohydrate absorption." *Clinics in Gastroenterology* 11: 17, 1982.

Hopfer, U. Digestion and absorption of basic nutritional constituents. T. M. Devlin (Ed.). *Textbook of Biochemistry with Clinical Correlations.* New York: Wiley-Liss, 1992, Chap. 26, p. 1059.

Ravich, W. J., and Bayless, T. M. "Carbohydrate absorption and malabsorption." *Clinics in Gastroenterology* 12: 335, 1983.

Semenza, G., and Auricchio, S. Small-intestinal disaccharidases. C. R. Scriver, A. L. Beaudet, W. S. Sly, and D. Valle (Eds.). *The Metabolic Basis of Inherited Disease.* New York: McGraw-Hill, 1989, Vol. II, Chap. 121, p. 2975.

Answer 16

a. Dermatan sulfate is a glycosaminoglycan containing L-iduronic acid, D-glucuronic acid, and N-acetylglucosamine, many of these residues being sulfated. The fact that your patient has difficulty removing the sulfate from the iduronate suggests that the defective enzyme is *iduronate sulfatase.*

b. See Figure A16-1.

Your patient has MUCOPOLYSACCHARIDOSIS II (HUNTER SYNDROME).

Reference
Neufeld, E. F., and Muenzer, J. The mucopolysaccharidoses. C. R. Scriver, A. L. Beaudet, W. S. Sly, and D. Valle (Eds.). *The Metabolic Basis of Inherited Disease.* New York: McGraw-Hill, 1989, Vol. II, Chap. 61, p. 1565.

Answer 17

a. Heparan sulfate is a glycosaminoglycan containing glucosamine, D-glucuronic acid, N-acetylglucosamine, and L-iduronic acid, many of these being sulfated. The fact that your patient has difficulty removing the sulfate from a glucosamine suggests that the defective enzyme is *heparan N-sulfatase*.

b. See Figure A17-1.

Your patient has MUCOPOLYSACCHARIDOSIS IIIA (SANFILIPPO A SYNDROME).

Reference
Neufeld, E. F., and Muenzer, J. The mucopolysaccharidoses. C. R. Scriver, A. L. Beaudet, W. S. Sly, and D. Valle (Eds.). *The Metabolic Basis of Inherited Disease.* New York: McGraw-Hill, 1989, Vol. II, Chap. 61, p. 1565.

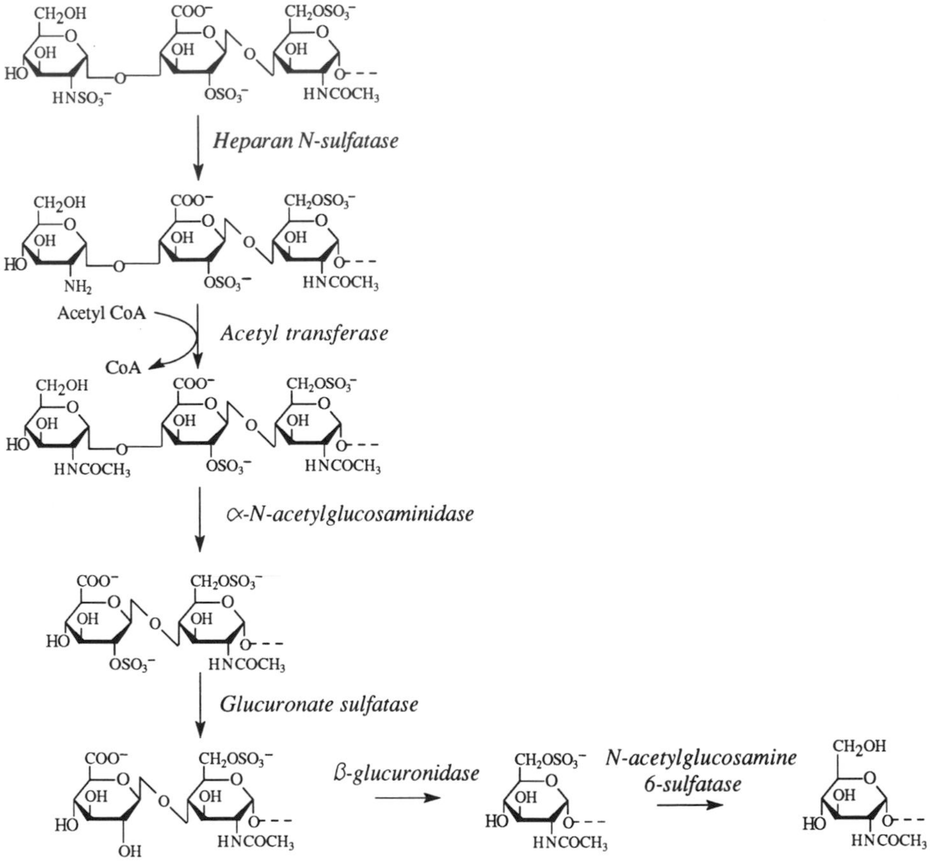

FIGURE A17-1. **Degradation of heparan sulfate.**

Answer 18

a. Keratan sulfate is a glycosaminoglycan consisting of galactose, *N*-acetylglucosamine, and glucose, some of these residues being sulfated. The fact that your patient has difficulty in removing sulfate from the galactose suggests that the defective enzyme is *galactose-6-sulfatase*.

b. See Figure A18-1.

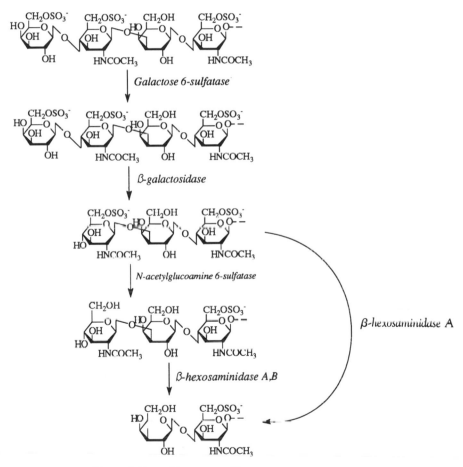

FIGURE A18-1. **Degradation of keratan sulfate.**

Your patient has MUCOPOLYSACCHARIDOSIS IVA (MORQUIO A SYNDROME).

Reference

Neufeld, E. F., and Muenzer, J. The mucopolysaccharidoses. C. R. Scriver, A. L. Beaudet, W. S. Sly, and D. Valle (Eds.). *The Metabolic Basis of Inherited Disease.* New York: McGraw-Hill, 1989, Vol. II, Chap. 61, p. 1565.

CHAPTER 4

Lipid Metabolism

Problem 19

Your patient is an 18-year-old girl with diarrhea following fatty meals. Her erythrocytes have a spiny shape. She exhibits ataxia and has an almost complete lack of chlomicra, very-low-density lipoproteins (VLDL), and low-density lipoproteins (LDL) in her blood. Her serum cholesterol level is very low. You do a liver biopsy and use a polyclonal antibody raised against the B-100 protein. With the antibody, you find that the B-100 protein and the B-48 protein are present in the cells at much lower than normal levels. You also determine that the level of mRNA for B-100 in these cells is very low.

a. What is the probable defect in your patient?

b. Why would you expect levels of high-density lipoprotein (HDL) to be normal in this patient?

Problem 20

Your patient is an infant who has great difficulty absorbing fats. He suffers severely from diarrhea. Biopsy reveals that his intestinal cells are full of fat droplets. He has no chylomicra in his plasma, even after meals. Treatment with a monoclonal antibody specific for B-48 shows that abnormally high levels of B-48 are present in his intestinal cells. Levels of B-100 are normal, however. You incubate the biopsy samples with [^{3}H]leucine and [^{14}C]mannose and purify the protein fraction. You then measure the ratio of ^{3}H to ^{14}C and find that it is 8.4, whereas in an equivalent sample from a normal person the ratio would be 3.0. Total protein synthesis in your patient's biopsy sample is about 31% less than that of a normal sample.

    a. What is the probable molecular defect in your patient?

    b. What is the significance of the high ^{3}H/^{14}C ratio in your patient?

    c. Why might it be helpful to feed this infant a diet with short- or medium-chain fatty acids?

Problem 21

Your patient comes from a family many of whose members have severe coronary arteriosclerosis, often appearing at relatively young ages. He has increased levels of both very-low-density lipoproteins (VLDL) and low-density lipoproteins (LDL) in his blood. You do a biopsy of his fibroblasts and find that the level of LDL receptor are normal. You then do a liver biopsy and find that the levels of mRNA coding for B-100 are very high.

a. What is the etiology of his disease?

b. You find that the level of B-100 mRNA in his intestinal cells is normal. Would you expect his chylomicron level to be normal? If so, why?

Problem 22

Your patient is a 59-year-old man with abdominal pain. Blood tests reveal very high concentrations of chylomicra, even after an overnight fast. Triglycerides are also elevated. He has a deficiency of apolipoprotein C-II.

a. Why would this deficiency cause a high level of chylomicra in his blood?

b. An as yet unexplained finding is that VLDL levels are normal in your patient. Why is this a surprise?

Problem 23

Your patient has high blood concentrations of cholesterol and triglycerides. He also has fatty eruptions on his elbows. You analyze his very-low-density lipoproteins (VLDL) and his chylomicra by isoelectric focusing. You find that apolipoprotein E from your patient is slightly more negative than apolipoprotein E from a normal person. You measure the binding of your patient's apolipoprotein E to cultured liver cells from a normal person and find that very little binding occurs. He has very low levels of low-density lipoproteins (LDL) in his blood. A liver biopsy shows that his level of LDL receptors is high.

a. How do these findings account for the high serum cholesterol level in your patient?

b. Why might your patient have high levels of LDL receptor?

c. Why would that cause low levels of circulating LDL?

Problem 24

Your patient has fatty deposits in his Achilles tendon. He exhibits tremors and is suffering from incontinence. He also has difficulty in swallowing. He has very high fecal and urinary levels of certain bile acid intermediates, specifically 5β-cholestane-3α, 7α, 12α, 23-tetrol, 5β-cholestane-3α, 7α, 12α, 25-tetrol, and 5β-cholestane-3α, 7α, 12α, 24, 25-pentol. You do a liver biopsy and culture the cells. You give the cells radioactive 7α-hydroxy-4-cholesten-3-one and find that production of 7α, 26-dihydroxy-4-cholesten-3-one is much lower than normal. Similarly, when you give the cells radioactive 5β-cholestane-3α, 7α-diol, you find that their production of 5β-cholestane-3α, 7α, 26-triol is very low.

a. Name the defective enzyme.

b. Show the pathway in which the conversion of 7α-hydroxy-4-cholesten-3-one to 7α, 26-dihydroxy-4-cholesten-3-one occurs.

c. If you gave your patient's liver cells radioactive 5β-cholestane-3α, 7α, 12α-triol would you expect to see increased or decreased production of 5β-cholestane-3α, 7α, 12α, 26-tetrol? Why?

Problem 25

Your patient is an 18-year-old boy with atherosclerosis of the coronary arteries. He also has fatty deposits on his tendons and under his skin in various places of his body. Analysis of his blood reveals high concentrations of steroids that cannot be made by mammals, including sitosterol and campesterol, as well as some stigmasterol. Biopsy of the fatty deposits reveals high amounts of sitosterol. One day he comes in for a blood test and you find relatively high concentrations of 22-dehydrocholesterol, brassicasterol, and 24-methylenecholesterol. It turned out that he had just had a meal of oysters Rockefeller and spaghetti with clam sauce. You now decide to put him on a diet.

a. In general, what sorts of foods should he avoid? (Don't just say oysters Rockefeller and spaghetti with clam sauce.)

b. Why do you tell him to eat butter rather than margarine, shrimp rather than scallops, and white bread rather than whole wheat? Why is it all right for him to eat cheese, eggs, and bacon?

c. What other treatment might you recommend?

Problem 26

Your patient is a 10-month-old child with poor muscle tone, seizures, and severe mental and physical retardation. Most fatty acids are metabolized normally in this child. However, very-long-chain fatty acids (over 24 carbons) are metabolized poorly. You do a liver biopsy and purify the peroxisomes from the liver cells. To the peroxisomes, you add radioactive stearate and measure its conversion to other products. The results are listed in Table P26-1 (expressed as the percentage of that obtained with a normal patient).

a. Name the defective enzyme. Write the reaction catalyzed by this enzyme. *Note:* The peroxisome does not do this the same way as does the mitochondrion.

b. What radioactive product would you expect to see accumulating if you add radioactive palmitate to your patient's peroxisomes?

TABLE P26-1

Product	Yield	Percent of Carbons in Fatty Acid Part of Product
Stearyl-CoA	180	18
trans-Δ^2-Enoyl-CoA	5	18
L-3-Hydroxyacyl-CoA	5	18
3-Ketoacyl-CoA	5	18
Palmityl-CoA	5	16

Problem 27

Your patient was a Harry Belafonte fan who was fascinated by the reference to "akee rice" in the song "Jamaica Farewell" and went to spend his vacation in Jamaica, gorging himself on cooked akee fruit. When he returned he smuggled some unripe akee fruit through customs and then ate some for lunch. The next day he was admitted to the hospital with severe vomiting and he expired shortly after telling you about his vacation. Analysis of his urine showed high levels of glutaric acid and 2-ethylmalonic acid. You obtain mitochondria from the liver cells and sonicate them (break them up into little fragments). You treat them with dichlorophenol indophenol (DCIP), an electron acceptor dye that changes color when it accepts an electron. You add NADH and find that the DCIP changes color as much as occurs in a mitochondrial preparation from a normal person. However, when you add glutaryl-CoA or palmityl-CoA, you find that the DCIP does not change color. Research in the library reveals that unripe akee fruit contains hypoglycin A, which our bodies metabolize to methylenecyclopropylacetyl-CoA.

a. What enzyme(s) do you think is/are inhibited by methylenecyclopropylacetyl-CoA?

b. If you were doing research on this disease, for example in an animal model, would you consider testing the therapeutic effect of riboflavin? Why, or why not?

Problem 28

Your patient is a 5-year-old girl with difficulty walking, talking, and hearing. Her plasma level of very-long-chain fatty acids is normal. The total bile acid concentration in her plasma is normal; however, the relative amounts are unusual: cholic acid and chenodeoxycholic acid levels are very low, while $3\alpha,7\alpha,12\alpha$-trihydroxy-5β-cholestan-26-oic acid and $3\alpha,7\alpha$-dihydroxy-5β-cholestan-26-oic acid are very high. You also find high levels of a dicarboxylic bile acid containing 29 carbons.

a. What is the defective enzyme? Write out the pathway in which this enzyme occurs.

b. In what organelle is this enzyme located?

Problem 29

Your patient is a 6-month-old child with an enlarged liver and a high fat content in his stool. He has anemia, frequent vomiting, and diarrhea and has a distended abdomen. X-rays show that his adrenal glands are full of calcium deposits. Biopsy of various tissues reveals that they are full of cholesteryl esters and triglycerides. You purify some lysosomes from his leukocytes and do an assay in which you add radioactive cholesterol esterified to palmitate and find that the release of free cholesterol is 0.5% of that which you would expect in a normal person.

a. Name the defective enzyme.

b. Further analysis shows that the enzyme is present in the leukocytes but is not located in lysosomes. What would you then say is the cause of the problem?

Problem 30

Your patient is a 2-year-old boy with mental and motor retardation. He has a cherry-red spot on his retina. He dies of pneumonia shortly after losing the ability to cough. Autopsy shows that his neurons are full of membranous inclusions near the nuclei. His brain contains very large quantities of ganglioside G_{M2}. Glycolipid G_{A2} concentrations are also elevated. You do an assay in which you purify your patient's lysosomes and add ganglioside G_{M2} labeled with radioactive N-acetylglucosamine. You find that release of N-acetylglucosamine does not occur. You also find that when you add radioactive glycolipid G_{A2}, no release of N-acetylglucosamine occurs. However, when you add synthetic substrates, you find that your patient's lysosomes are normal in their ability to release N-acetylglucosamine from these substrates. You now add ganglioside G_{M2} in the presence of detergent and find that your patient's lysosomes are now able to cause normal release of N-acetylglucosamine. You get the same result when you add glycolipid G_{A2}.

    a. What reaction is defective in your patient?

    b. Name the defective protein.

    c. What would you say is the role of this protein?

Answer 19

a. The protein moieties of lipoproteins are referred to as *apolipoproteins;* these are classified into the following families: apolipoproteins A, B, C, D, E, F, and G. Several of these families are further subdivided. The different types of lipoproteins differ in the nature of their component apolipoproteins. Thus the proteins of chylomicra consist of 60 to 65% apolipoprotein C, 20 to 22% B, 5% E, 1% D, and 0 to 3% A. Those of VLDL are 40 to 50% apolipoprotein B, 35 to 40% C, 5 to 10% E, and 0 to 3% A. Those of LDL are 95 to 100% apolipoprotein B, 0 to 5% C, and trace amounts of A. The data obtained with the antibody suggest that there are abnormally low amounts of apolipoprotein B in your patient. Since apolipoprotein B is a major constituent of chylomicra, VLDL, and LDL, it is not surprising that all of these are low.

Actually, several forms of apolipoprotein B exist. The two most important are designated B-100 (MW 549,000) and B-48 (MW 264,000) of 4536 and 2152 residues, respectively. B-100 is the major species of apolipoprotein B in LDL and B-48 is the major species in chylomicra. The fact that the antibody against B-100 is polyclonal suggests that it might bind to several fragments of B-100, including B-48, and would imply that all of these are low in your patient. The fact that B-48 levels are low is consistent with this notion. This is an intriguing conclusion since it appears that B-48 and B-100 are encoded in the same gene and that in the transcription of B-48 a stop codon replaces Gln^{2153} in B-100. The fact that mRNA levels for B-100 are low suggests that the defect is one of transcription. Perhaps a promoter or enhancer element in your patient is defective and this could conceivably affect the transcription of both B-100 and B-48.

b. The apolipoproteins of HDL consists of 90 to 95% apolipoprotein A, 4 to 6% C, 0 to 2% B, 0 to 2% D, and traces of F and G. The fact that so little of HDL consists of apolipoprotein B implies that a defect in its synthesis would have little effect on HDL levels.

Your patient has ABETALIPOPROTEINEMIA.

References

Kane, J. P., and Havel, R. J. Disorders of the biogenesis and secretion of lipoproteins containing the B apolipoproteins. C. R. Scriver, A. L. Beaudet, W. S. Sly, and D.

Valle (Eds.). *The Metabolic Basis of Inherited Disease.* New York: McGraw-Hill, 1989, Vol. I, Chap. 44B, p. 1139.

Schultz, R. M., and Liebman, M. N. Proteins I: composition and structure. T. M. Devlin (Ed.). *Textbook of Biochemistry with Clinical Correlations.* New York: Wiley-Liss, 1992, Chap. 2, p. 25.

Answer 20

a. Your patient lacks chylomicra, suggesting that he may have a problem in the synthesis or secretion of one of the constituent apolipoproteins of chylomicra. These consist of 60 to 65% apolipoprotein C, 20 to 22% B, 5% E, 1% D, and 0 to 3% A. In chylomicra, the major form of apolipoprotein B is B-48. The fact that abnormally high concentrations of B-48 are found in the intestinal cells suggests that the protein is made but not secreted. If so, your patient would not be able to make chylomicra, which normally have large amounts of B-48.

b. Your patient's protein synthesis is somewhat suppressed. However, much less mannose is being incorporated into your patient's proteins. In other words, not only is your patient making less protein, he has trouble glycosylating the proteins he does make. The low levels of glycosylation of the proteins made by your patient's intestinal cells implies that the defect is in the glycosylation of B-48, which in turn inhibits its secretion and the production of chylomicra.

c. Short- and medium-chain fatty acids do not need chylomicra for absorption. Hence, even with a low level of chylomicra, your patient would still be able to obtain the fatty acids he needs.

Your patient has HYPOBETALIPOPROTEINEMIA.

References

Kane, J. P., and Havel, R. J. Disorders of the biogenesis and secretion of lipoproteins containing the B apolipoproteins. C. R. Scriver, A. L. Beaudet, W. S. Sly, and D. Valle (Eds.). *The Metabolic Basis of Inherited Disease.* New York: McGraw-Hill, 1989, Vol. I, Chap. 44B, p. 1139.

Levy, E., Marcel, Y., Deckelbaum, R. J., Milne, R., Lepage, G., Seidman, E., Bendayan, M., and Roy, C. C. Intestinal apoB synthesis, lipids, and lipoproteins in chylomicron retention disease. *J. Lipid Res.* 28: 1263, 1987.

Answer 21

a. Your patient has elevated levels of VLDL and LDL. One possible explanation would be that there are too few LDL receptors to absorb the VLDL and LDL, but the levels of LDL receptor are normal. Therefore, there must be high production of LDL, or specifically of one or more of its constituent apolipoproteins. The elevated mRNA for B-100 implies that the defect is excessive synthesis in the liver of apolipoprotein B-100, a major component of LDL and VLDL. The precise cause of this disease is not yet known, but recent work suggests that the defective gene may be located on chromosome 11.

b. You would expect the chylomicron levels to be normal, because the B-100 mRNA level in the intestine is normal. B-48 is a constituent of chylomicra; B-48 appears to be an alternatively transcribed form of B-100; it is likely that if B-100 levels are normal in the intestine, B-48 levels will also be normal. Since B-48 is a major constituent of chylomicra, the latter would also be present in normal amounts.

Your patient has FAMILIAL COMBINED HYPERLIPIDEMIA (FAMILIAL MULTIPLE-TYPE HYPERLIPOPROTEINEMIA).

References

Kane, J. P., and Havel, R. J. Disorders of the biogenesis and secretion of lipoproteins containing the B apolipoproteins. C. R. Scriver, A. L. Beaudet, W. S. Sly, and D. Valle (Eds.). *The Metabolic Basis of Inherited Disease.* New York: McGraw-Hill, 1989, Vol. I, Chap. 44B, p. 1139.

Wojciechowski, A. P., Farrall, M., Cullen, P., Wilson, T. M. E., Bayliss, J. D., Farren, B., Griffin, B. A., Caslake, M. J., Packard, C. J., Shepherd, J., Thakker, R., and Scott, J. Familial combined hyperlipidaemia linked to the apolipoprotein AI-CIII-AIV gene cluster on chromosome 11q23-q24. *Nature* 349: 161, 1991.

Answer 22

a. Chylomicra contain several apolipoproteins. Of these, 60 to 65% consist of apolipoprotein C. The latter consists of three species: apo C-I, apo C-II, and apo C-III, which account, respectively, for 5 to 10%, 15%, and 40% of the total apolipoproteins in chylomicra. At first glance it is surprising that a defect in apolipoprotein C-II would cause an increase in the chylomicron level, since this protein is a constituent of chylomicra. The fact that it does, however, suggests that apolipoprotein C-II must be playing another role in chylomicra. This is indeed the case. Apolipoprotein C-II is an activator of the enzyme lipoprotein lipase, an enzyme that cleaves triglycerides in both chylomicra and VLDL. In so doing, lipoprotein lipase converts the chylomicra into remnants that are degraded by the liver. In the absence of apolipoprotein C-II, the activity of lipoprotein lipase will be low and hence degradation of chylomicra will not occur, leading to high concentrations of chylomicra in the blood.

b. Digestion of VLDL by lipoprotein lipase should be inhibited as well if the activity of lipoprotein lipase is low. It is not clear, therefore, why VLDL concentrations are normal.

Your patient has CHYLOMICRONEMIA.

Reference

Brunzell, J. D. Familial lipoprotein lipase deficiency and other causes of the chylomicronemia syndrome. C. R. Scriver, A. L. Beaudet, W. S. Sly, and D. Valle (Eds.). *The Metabolic Basis of Inherited Disease.* New York: McGraw-Hill, 1989, Vol. I. Chap. 45, p. 1165.

Answer 23

a. Apolipoprotein E is a constituent of chylomicra and VLDL. The role of apolipoprotein E is to connect the chylomicra and VLDL with a receptor in liver cells. Your patient's abnormal apolipoprotein E is unable to make this connection; hence the chylomicra and VLDL do not interact with these receptors and may end up being taken up by macrophages; these macrophages may in turn contribute to these fatty eruptions in your patient.

b. The cells are starved for cholesterol because they are unable to take up the cholesterol carried by chylomicra and VLDL. Their response to this is to make more LDL receptor so as to take up LDL-cholesterol.

c. The excess LDL receptor removes the LDL in the blood.

Your patient has TYPE III HYPERLIPOPROTEINEMIA (DYSBETALIPOPROTEINEMIA).

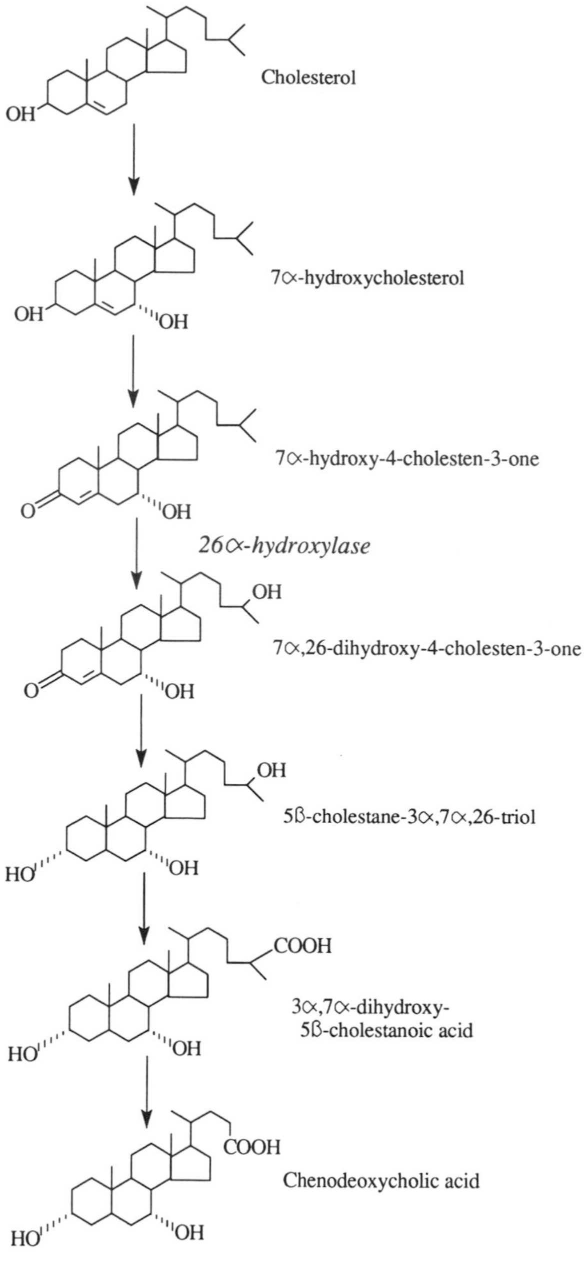

FIGURE A24-1. **Conversion of cholesterol to chenodeoxycholic acid.**

Reference

Mahley, R. W., and Rall, A. C. Type III hyperlipoproteinemia (dysbetalipoproteinemia): the role of apolipoprotein E in normal and abnormal lipoprotein metabolism. C. R. Scriver, A. L. Beaudet, W. S. Sly, and D. Valle (Eds.). *The Metabolic Basis of Inherited Disease.* New York: McGraw-Hill, 1989, Vol. I, Chap. 47, p. 1195.

Answer 24

a. The missing enzyme is the one that converts 7α-hydroxy-4-cholesten-3-one to 7α,26-dihydroxy-4-cholesten-3-one. This is the mitochondrial 26α-hydroxylase.

b. See Figure A24.1. The reaction catalyzed by 26α-hydroxylase is indicated in the pathway.

c. If you gave your patient's liver cells radioactive 5β-cholestane-3α,7α,12α-triol, you would expect to see decreased production of 5β-cholestane-3α,7α,12α,26-tetrol because 26α-hydroxylase is needed to hydroxylate carbon 26.

Your patient has CEREBROTENDINOUS XANTHOMATOSIS.

References

Björkheim, I., and Skrede, S. Familial diseases with storage of sterols other than cholesterol: cerebrotendinous xanthomatosis and phytosterolemia. C. R. Scriver, A. L. Beaudet, W. S. Sly, and D. Valle (Eds.). *The Metabolic Basis of Inherited Disease.* New York: McGraw-Hill, 1989, Vol. I, Chap. 51, p. 1283.

Salen, G., and Mosbach, E. H. The metabolism of sterols and bile acids in cerebrotendinous xanthomatosis. P. P. Nair and D. Kritchevsky (Eds.). *The Bile Acids: Chemistry, Physiology, and Metabolism.* New York: Plenum Press, 1971, Vol. 3, Chap. 6, p. 115.

Answer 25

a. He should avoid vegetable oils of all kinds and molluscs. These are rich in the rather unusual steroids shown in Figure A25-1.

b. He needs to avoid vegetable oils, which occur in seeds, kernels, and margarine but not in butter. He must stay away from shellfish sterols,

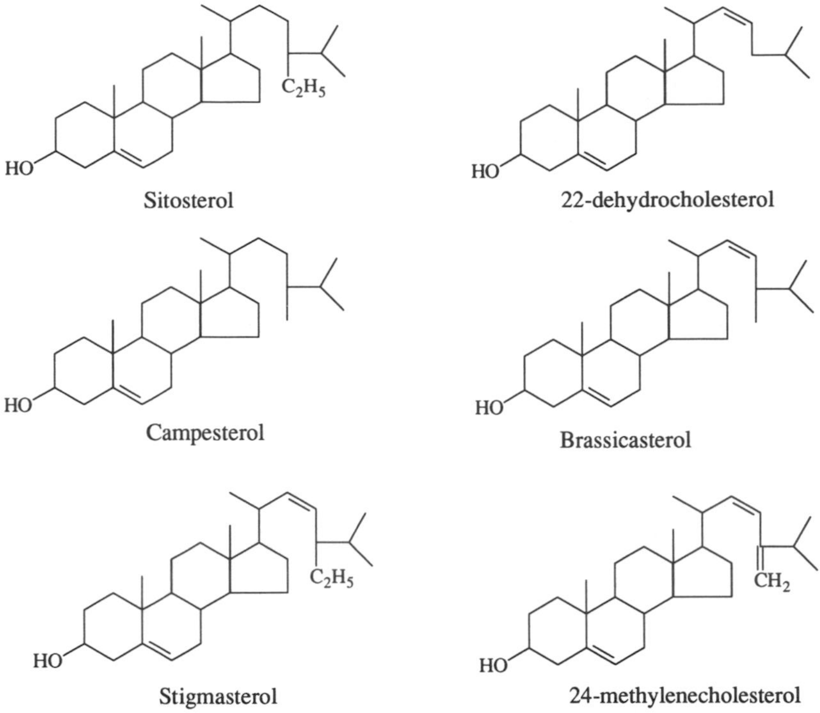

FIGURE A25-1. **Structures of some plant and mollusc steroids. Plant steroids are shown on the left and mollusc steroids on the right.**

which are found in molluscs but not in crustaceans. Refined flour is fine. Animal fats are all right for this patient; at least, there is no reason to think otherwise.

c. The fundamental cause of this disease is unknown, but it is thought to be related to increased intestinal absorption of these plant and molluscan steroids. One treatment might be to give your patient cholestyramine, a substance which is used as a treatment for individuals with elevated cholesterol. Cholestyramine is a resin which complexes with bile acids in the intestine; this complex is then excreted in the feces. By blocking bile acid reabsorption, cholestyramine forces a shift in the body's cholesterol metabolism so that more cholesterol goes into bile acid synthesis. The effect on the liver is to increase LDL receptor synthesis which then lowers the blood level of LDL-cholesterol. Cholestyramine should also be able to prevent absorption of the plant and mollusc sterols and indeed has been successfully used to treat this disease.

Your patient has PHYTOSTEROLEMIA.

References

Ast, M., and Frishman, W. H. "Bile acid sequestrants." *J. Clin. Pharmacol.* 30: 99, 1990.

Belamarich, P. F., Deckelbaum, R. J., Starc, T. J., Dobrin, B. E., Tint, G. S., and Salen, G. "Response to diet and cholestyramine in a patient with sitosterolemia." *Pediatrics* 86: 977, 1990.

Björkheim, I., and Skrede, S. Familial diseases with storage of sterols other than choles-terol: cerebrotendinous xanthomatosis and phytosterolemia. C. R. Scriver, A. L. Beaudet, W. S. Sly, and D. Valle (Eds.). *The Metabolic Basis of Inherited Disease.* New York: McGraw-Hill, 1989, Vol. I, Chap. 51, p. 1283.

Salen, G., Shefer, S., Nguyen, L., Ness, G. C., Tint, G. S., and Shore, V. Sitostero-lemia. *J. Lipid Res.* 33: 945, 1992.

Answer 26

a. Unlike mitochondria, peroxisomes are able to oxidize very-long-chain fatty acids. The fact that your patient can oxidize other fatty acids suggests that his mitochondria are working normally but that there is a defect in the peroxisomes. When the peroxisomes are purified, they are unable to convert stearate into palmityl-CoA, which means that they are unable to go through a full cycle of β oxidation. Obviously, one of the enzymes in the pathway is missing. Since the stearoyl-CoA accumulates while the subsequent compounds are present in much lower quantities, the defect must be in the enzyme that converts stearoyl-CoA into *trans*-Δ^2-enoyl-CoA; this enzyme is *acyl-CoA oxidase.* The peroxisomal β-oxidation pathway is shown in Figure A26-1.

b. If you give the peroxisomes radioactive palmitate, you would expect the same type of metabolic block. Since the peroxisomal

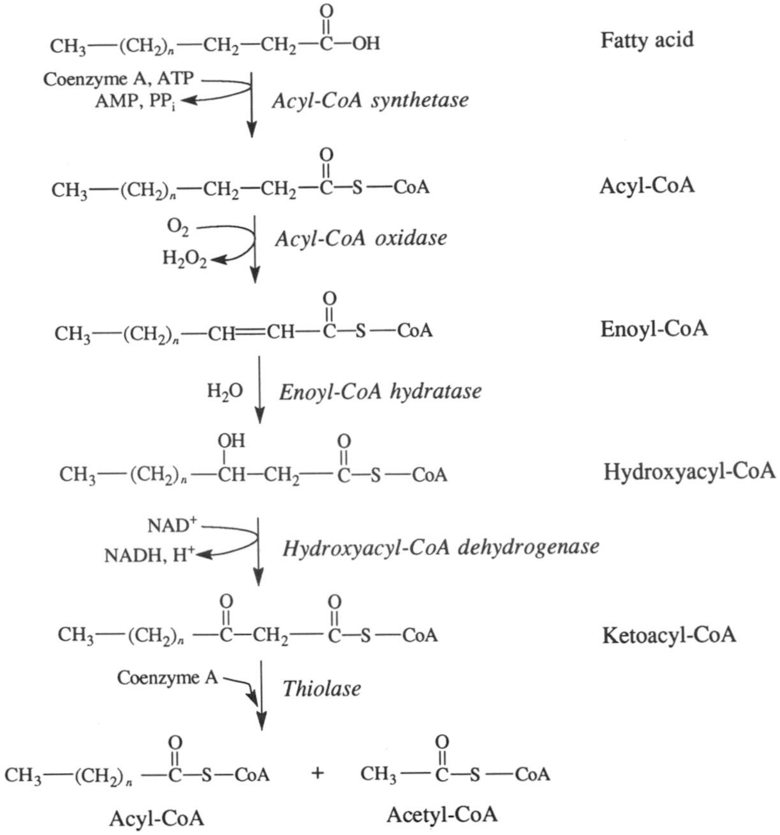

$$CH_3 \!-\! (CH_2)_n \!-\! CH_2 \!-\! CH_2 \!-\! \overset{\overset{\displaystyle O}{\|}}{C} \!-\! OH \qquad \text{Fatty acid}$$

Coenzyme A, ATP
AMP, PP$_i$ — *Acyl-CoA synthetase*

$$CH_3 \!-\! (CH_2)_n \!-\! CH_2 \!-\! CH_2 \!-\! \overset{\overset{\displaystyle O}{\|}}{C} \!-\! S \!-\! CoA \qquad \text{Acyl-CoA}$$

O$_2$
H$_2$O$_2$ — *Acyl-CoA oxidase*

$$CH_3 \!-\! (CH_2)_n \!-\! CH \!=\! CH \!-\! \overset{\overset{\displaystyle O}{\|}}{C} \!-\! S \!-\! CoA \qquad \text{Enoyl-CoA}$$

H$_2$O — *Enoyl-CoA hydratase*

$$CH_3 \!-\! (CH_2)_n \!-\! \overset{\overset{\displaystyle OH}{|}}{CH} \!-\! CH_2 \!-\! \overset{\overset{\displaystyle O}{\|}}{C} \!-\! S \!-\! CoA \qquad \text{Hydroxyacyl-CoA}$$

NAD$^+$
NADH, H$^+$ — *Hydroxyacyl-CoA dehydrogenase*

$$CH_3 \!-\! (CH_2)_n \!-\! \overset{\overset{\displaystyle O}{\|}}{C} \!-\! CH_2 \!-\! \overset{\overset{\displaystyle O}{\|}}{C} \!-\! S \!-\! CoA \qquad \text{Ketoacyl-CoA}$$

Coenzyme A — *Thiolase*

$$CH_3 \!-\! (CH_2)_n \!-\! \overset{\overset{\displaystyle O}{\|}}{C} \!-\! S \!-\! CoA \quad + \quad CH_3 \!-\! \overset{\overset{\displaystyle O}{\|}}{C} \!-\! S \!-\! CoA$$

Acyl-CoA   Acetyl-CoA

FIGURE A26-1. **Peroxisomal β-oxidation pathway.**

acyl-CoA oxidase is defective, you would see an accumulation of palmityl-CoA.

References

Lazarow, P. B., and Moser, H. W. Disorders of peroxisome biogenesis. C. R. Scriver, A. L. Beaudet, W. S. Sly, and D. Valle (Eds.). *The Metabolic Basis of Inherited Disease.* New York: McGraw-Hill, 1989, Vol. II, Chap. 57, p. 1479.

Wanders, R. J. A., Van Roermund, C. W. T., Schutgens, R. B. H., Barth, P. G., Heymans, H. S. A., Van den Bosch, H., and Tager, J. M. The inborn errors of peroxisomal β-oxidation: a review. *J. Inherit. Metab. Dis.* 13: 4, 1990.

Answer 27

a. Electron transport starting with NADH seems to be normal with your patient. However, electron transport starting with glutaryl-CoA or palmityl-CoA is not normal. The hypoglycin A from the unripe akee fruit is metabolized to methylenecyclopropylacetyl-CoA, which may interfere with an enzyme involved in this pathway of electron transport. These enzymes are either *electron transfer flavoprotein (ETF)* or *ETF ubiquinone oxidoreductase* or an *acyl-CoA dehydrogenase*. The structures of hypoglycin A and methylenecyclopropylacetyl-CoA are shown in Figure A27-1.

b. Riboflavin is a cofactor of ETF. It is thought that methylenecyclo-propylacetyl-CoA may react covalently with the flavin moiety of ETF and inactivate it. It appears to be a "suicide" inactivator. First, the acyl-CoA dehydrogenase oxidizes the methylenecyclopropylacetyl-CoA, which then proceeds to react covalently with the flavin, thereby inactivating the enzyme. It is likely that extra riboflavin might compensate for the effect of the poison. The hypothetical reaction scheme for inactivation is shown in Figure A27-2. Methylenecyclopropylacetyl-CoA is particularly inhibitory of the medium- and short-chain acyl-CoA dehydrogenases and of the isovaleryl-CoA dehydrogenase.

Your patient had JAMAICAN VOMITING SICKNESS.

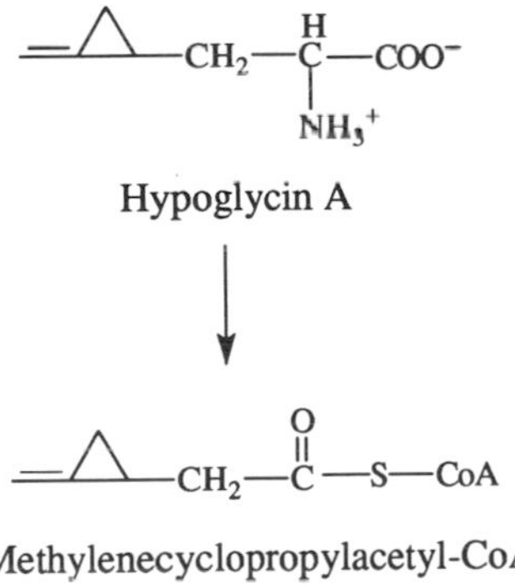

FIGURE A27-1. **Conversion of hypoglycin A to methylenecyclopropylacetyl-CoA.**

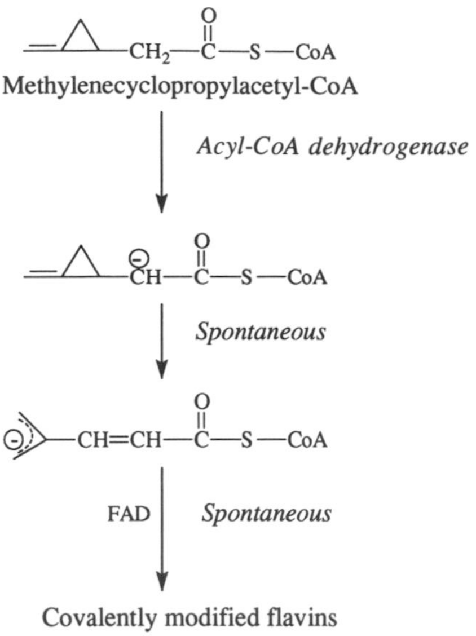

Methylenecyclopropylacetyl-CoA

Acyl-CoA dehydrogenase

Spontaneous

FAD | *Spontaneous*

Covalently modified flavins

FIGURE A27-2. **Possible inactivation of acyl-CoA dehydrogenase by methylenecyclopropylacetyl-CoA.**

References

Ghisla, S., Melde, K., Zeller, H. D., and Boschert, W. Mechanisms of enzyme inhibition by hypoglycin, methylenecyclopropylglycine and their metabolites. K. Tanaka and P. M. Coates (Eds.). *Fatty Acid Oxidation: Clinical, Biochemical, and Molecular Aspects* (Progress in Clinical and Biological Research, v. 321). New York: Alan R. Liss, p. 185.

Ikeda, Y., and Tanaka, T. Selective inactivation of various acyl-CoA dehydrogenases by (methylenecyclopropyl)acetyl-CoA. *Biochim. Biophys. Acta* 1038: 216, 1990.

Tanaka, K., and Ikeda, Y. Hypoglycin and Jamaican vomiting sickness. K. Tanaka and P. M. Coates (Eds.). *Fatty Acid Oxidation: Clinical, Biochemical, and Molecular Aspects* (Progress in Clinical and Biological Research, v. 321). New York: Alan R. Liss, 1990, p. 167.

Wenz, A., Thorpe, C., and Ghisla, S. Inactivation of general acyl-CoA dehydrogenase from pig kidney by a metabolite of hypolycin A. *J. Biol. Chem.* 256: 9809, 1981.

Answer 28

a. There is clearly a problem in the metabolism of bile salts. The fact that total bile salt levels are normal suggests that the defect cannot be early in the pathway going from cholesterol to the bile salts. Cholic acid is made from $3\alpha,7\alpha,12\alpha$-trihydroxy-5β-cholestan-26-oic acid and chenodeoxycholic acid is made from $3\alpha,7\alpha$-dihydroxy-5β-cholestan-26-oic acid. Hence the missing enzyme must be one that catalyzes one of the reactions in their biosynthetic pathway. The pathway consists of five enzymes and is shown in Figures A28-1 and A28-2. Three of these enzymes (enoyl-CoA hydratase, 3-hydroxyacyl-CoA dehydrogenase, and 3-oxoacyl-CoA thiolase) also catalyze oxidation of very-long-chain fatty acids. Since we are told that the very-long-chain fatty acids are present in normal quantities, the defective enzyme cannot be one of these three. This leaves two enzymes, which are both unique to the synthesis of cholic acid and chenodeoxycholic acid: microsomal $3\alpha,7\alpha,12\alpha$-trihydroxy-5β-cholestan-26-oyl-CoA synthetase and $3\alpha,7\alpha,12\alpha$-trihydroxy-5β-cholestan-26-oyl-CoA oxidase. One of these must be defective to account for your results.

At this point the elevated level of the 29-carbon dicarboxylic acid enters the picture. Even if the precise structure cannot as yet be characterized, it is probably made by elongation of a 27-carbon bile acid such as $3\alpha,7\alpha,12\alpha$-trihydroxy-5β-cholestan-26-oic acid. The elongation step requires that the substrate ($3\alpha,7\alpha,12\alpha$-trihydroxy-5β-cholestan-26-oic acid) be attached to coenzyme A. Hence if this 29-carbon bile acid is being made at a normal or higher rate, the enzyme that attaches $3\alpha,7\alpha,12\alpha$-trihydroxy-5β-cholestan-26-oic acid to coenzyme A must be present. Thus the defective enzyme is $3\alpha,7\alpha,12\alpha$-trihydroxy-5β-cholestan-26-oyl-CoA oxidase.

b. This enzyme is located in the *peroxisomes.*

References

Björkheim, I. Mechanism of bile acid biosynthesis is mammalian liver. H. Danielsson and J. Sjövall (Eds.). *Sterols and Bile Acids*. Amsterdam: Elsevier, 1985, Chap. 9, p. 231.

Cass, O. W., Williams, G. C., and Hanson, R. F. Competitive inhibition of side chain oxidation of $3\alpha,7\alpha$-dihydroxy-5β-cholestan-26-oic acid by $3\alpha,7\alpha,12\alpha$-tridroxy-5β-cholestan-26-oic acid in the hamster. *J. Lipid Res.* 21: 186, 1980.

Christensen, E., Van Eldere, J., Brandt, N. J., Schutgens, R. B. H., Wanders, R. J. A., and Eyssen, H. J. A new peroxisomal disorder: di- and trihydroxycholestanaemia due to a presumed trihydroxycholestanoyl-CoA oxidase deficiency. *J. Inherit. Metab. Dis.* 13: 363, 1990.

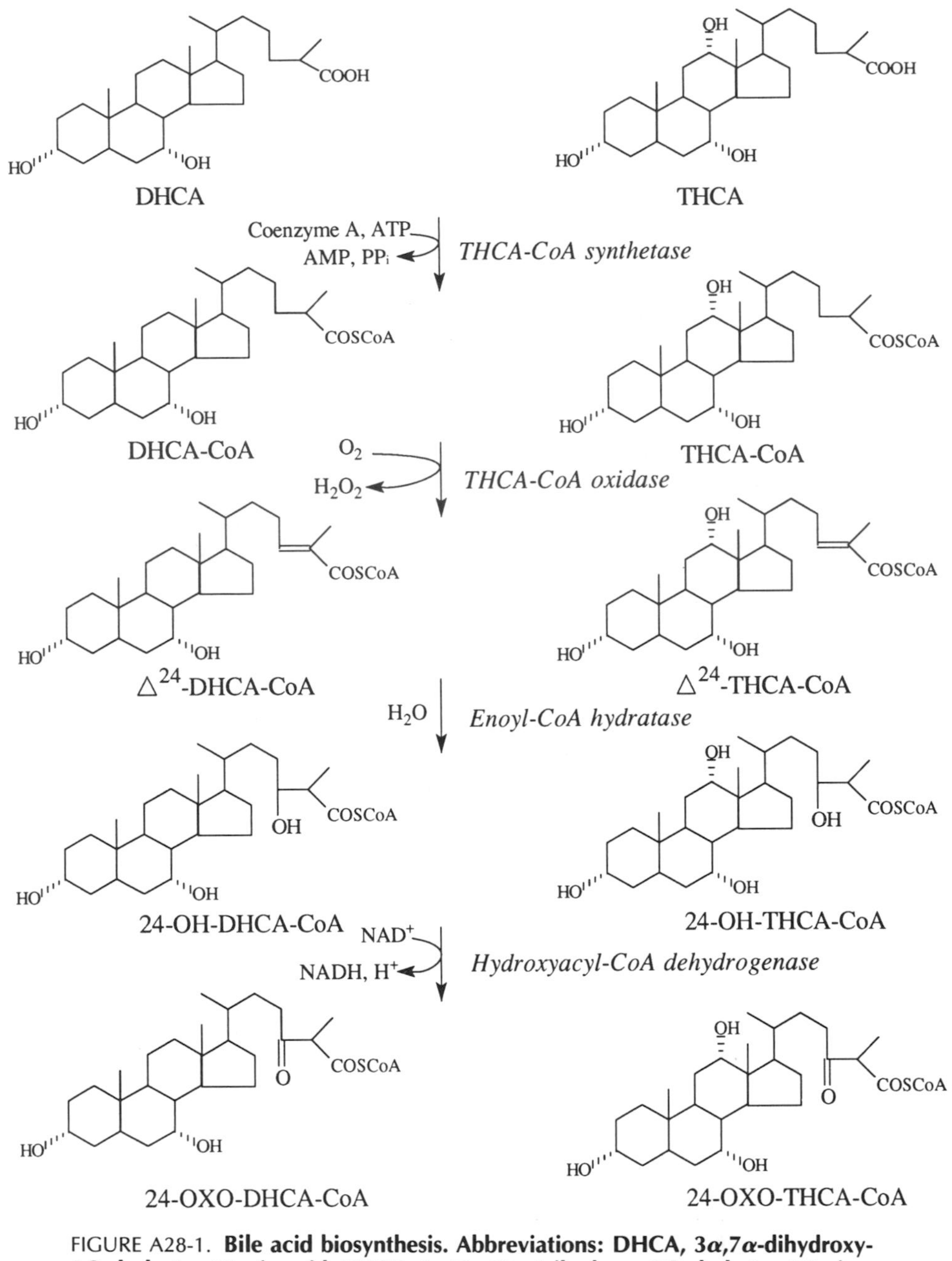

FIGURE A28-1. **Bile acid biosynthesis. Abbreviations: DHCA, $3\alpha,7\alpha$-dihydroxy-5β-cholestan-26-oic acid; THCA, $3\alpha,7\alpha,12\alpha$-trihydroxy-5β-cholestan-26-oic acid.**

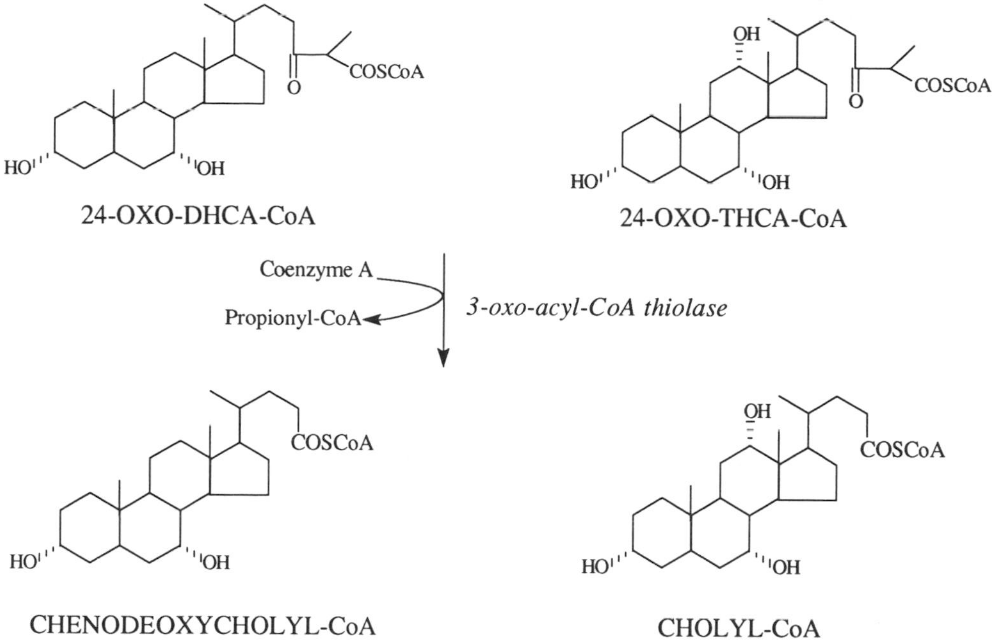
COSCoA
HO
OH
24-OXO-DHCA-CoA
OH
COSCoA
HO
OH
24-OXO-THCA-CoA
Coenzyme A
Propionyl-CoA
3-oxo-acyl-CoA thiolase
COSCoA
HO
OH
OH
COSCoA
HO
OH
CHENODEOXYCHOLYL-CoA
CHOLYL-CoA

FIGURE A28-2. **Bile acid biosynthesis (continued). Abbreviations are the same as in Figure 28-1.**

Wanders, R. J. A., Van Roermund, C. W. T., Schutgens, R. B. H., Barth, P. G., Heymans, H. S. A., Van den Bosch, H., and Tager, J. M. The inborn errors of peroxisomal β-oxidation: a review. *J. Inherit. Metab. Dis.* 13: 4, 1990.

Answer 29

a. In lysosomes cholesteryl esters are cleaved to release free cholesterol and a fatty acid. In the case of your patient, the lysosomes are unable to do this reaction. Hence the defective enzyme is *lysosomal acid lipase,* which is the one that normally carries out this cleavage (Figure A29-1).

b. If the enzyme is present in the leukocytes but not in their lysosomes, the problem must be in the targeting or transport of the enzyme. In other words, either the enzyme cannot be targeted to the lysosome

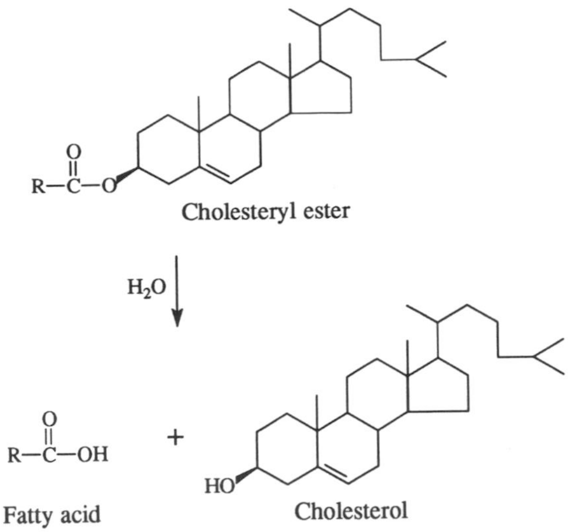

Cholesteryl ester

H_2O

R—C—OH   +

Fatty acid   Cholesterol

FIGURE A29-1. **Lysosomal acid lipase reaction.**

or else the transportation system for getting the enzyme into the lysosome is at fault.

Reference

Schmitz, G., and Assman, G. Acid lipase deficiency: Wolman disease and cholesteryl ester storage disease. C. R. Scriver, A. L. Beaudet, W. S. Sly, and D. Valle (Eds.). *The Metabolic Basis of Inherited Disease.* New York: McGraw-Hill, 1989, Vol. II, Chap. 64, p. 1623.

Answer 30

a. Your patient appears unable to remove N-acetylglucosamine from either ganglioside G_{M2} or glycolipid G_{A2}. This reaction is catalyzed by *hexosaminidase* A. The reaction is shown in Figure A30-1.

b. The fact that your patient's lysosomes can act on a synthetic substrate suggests that the enzyme hexosaminidase A is present and potentially functional in your patient. The fact that addition of detergent allows the reaction to occur suggests the same thing. There is a protein called G_{M2} *activator* which releases ganglioside G_{M2} from the membrane

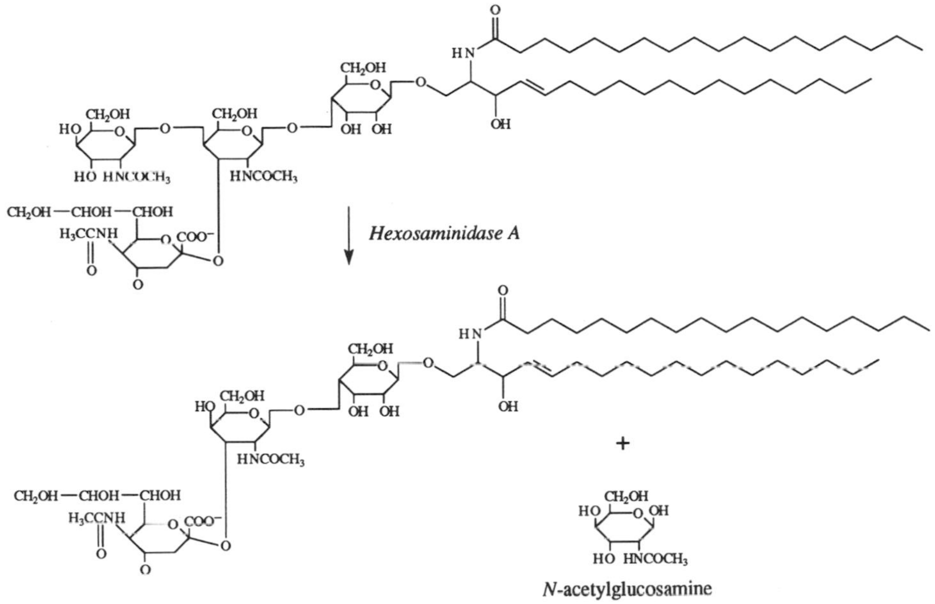

FIGURE A30-1. **Cleavage of ganglioside G_{M2} by hexosaminidase A.**

and allows it to be degraded by hexosaminidase A. This activator must be the defective protein. Interestingly, there is another activator protein involved in the metabolism of ganglioside G_{M1}.

c. Since the defective protein can be replaced by a detergent, it must itself act like a detergent and disrupt the membranes to permit release of ganglioside G_{M2}.

References

Li, Y.-T., and Li, S.-C. Activator proteins for the catabolism of glycosphingolipids. R. W. Ledeen, Yu, R. K., Rapport, M. M., and Suzuki, K. (Eds.). *Ganglioside Structure, Function, and Biomedical Potential* (Advances in Experimental Medicine and Biology, v. 174). New York: Plenum Press, 1984, p. 213.

Sandhoff, K., Conzelmann, E., Neufeld, E. F., Kaback, M. M., and Suzuki, K. The G_{M2} gangliosidoses. C. R. Scriver, A. L. Beaudet, W. S. Sly, and D. Valle (Eds.). *The Metabolic Basis of Inherited Disease.* New York: McGraw-Hill, 1989, Vol. II, Chap. 72, p. 1807.

CHAPTER 5

Vitamins

Problem 31

Your patient is an infant who exhibits recurrent vomiting, respiratory distress, and failure to thrive. He has a high serum level of both the D- and L-forms of methylmalonic acid. Circulating levels of vitamin B_{12} are normal. His condition does not respond to vitamin B_{12} injections. You culture some of his fibroblasts, prepare a cell-free extract, and measure the ability of the extract to carry out certain reactions when particular forms of cobalamin are added. You obtain the results shown in Table P31-1.

a. Name the defective enzyme.

b. Write out the pathway in which this enzyme occurs.

TABLE P31-1

Valence of Cobalt in Cobalamin	L-Methylmalonyl CoA → Succinate	Homocysteine → Methionine
+3	Reaction does not occur	Reaction is normal
+1	Reaction is normal	Not determined

Problem 32

You have two patients, both of whom appear to have pernicious anemia (neurological problems, methylmalonic acidemia, anemia). You find, however, that the level of intrinsic factor is normal in their intestines. Serum cobalamin levels are normal. You do liver biopsies and you find that cobalamin levels in their liver cells are extremely low. You decide to do the following experiment, in which you use your patients' liver cells and also liver cells from a normal person. You also collect serum from your patients and from a normal person. You have used immunoaffinity chromatography to remove all the cobalamin from the serum samples. You then try various combinations of the cells and sera and add radioactive cobalamin; you measure the amount of cobalamin incorporated into the cells. The results are shown in Table P32-1.

a. Name the defective protein in patient 1.

b. What is the probable defect in patient 2?

TABLE P32-1

Source of Cells	Source of Serum	Incorporation of Radioactive Cobalamin into Cells (% of normal)
Normal person	Normal person	100
Normal person	Patient 1	5
Patient 1	Normal person	100
Patient 1	Patient 1	5
Normal person	Patient 2	100
Patient 2	Normal person	5
Patient 2	Patient 2	5
Patient 2	Patient 1	5
Patient 1	Patient 2	100

Problem 33

Your patient is a 5-month-old girl with breathing problems, lethargy, and metabolic acidosis. Her urine shows elevated levels of β-hydroxypropionate, methylcitrate, β-methylcrotonylglycine, and other organic acids. You culture her fibroblasts and prepare a cell-free extract. To this you add radioactive propionyl-CoA and find that very little methylmalonyl-CoA is produced. You add radioactive pyruvate and find that very little oxaloacetate is produced. You add radioactive 3-methylcrotonyl-CoA and find that very little 3-methylglutaconyl-CoA is produced. The concentration of biotin in these cells is normal. Finally, you add radioactive biotin and measure how much gets incorporated into proteins; you find that incorporation into protein is much lower than normal.

a. Name the defective enzyme and describe the reaction catalyzed by the enzyme.

b. Describe the cycle of which this enzyme is a part.

c. Dietary biotin can help this disease, but not in every case. Why might it help in some cases and not in others?

Answer 31

a. Derivatives of vitamin B_{12} (cobalamin) participate as cofactors in a few metabolic reactions. One of these, catalyzed by *homocysteine methyltransferase*, requires methylcobalamin, and converts homocysteine to methionine in the cytosol. The other, occurring in the mitochondria, is catalyzed by *methylmalonyl CoA mutase*; this enzyme converts L-methylmalonyl-CoA into succinyl-CoA, which is then metabolized to succinate. The enzyme requires deoxyadenosylcobalamin. In both methylcobalamin and deoxyadenosylcobalamin the cobalt atom must be in the $+1$ oxidation state, although in dietary cobalamin the cobalt is in the $+3$ oxidation state.

Table P31-1 shows that the cytosolic reaction (conversion of homocysteine to methionine) occurs normally in the extract even when the cobalamin is in the $+3$ state. This means that the cytosolic cobalamin reductase, which converts cobalamin from the $+3$ to the $+1$ state, must be functioning normally and that the methylation of the cobalamin is normal. In contrast, the mitochondrial reaction (methylmalonyl-CoA mutase) does not work with the cobalamin in the $+3$ state. The fact that it is normal with cobalamin in the $+1$ state suggests that there is no problem with cobalamin getting inside the mitochondria or with the addition of the adenosyl group. Therefore, the defect must be in the mitochondrial *cobalamin reductase*.

b. Cobalamin reductase converts cobalamin (III) to cobalamin (II) and then to cobalamin (I) (Figure A31-1).

Your patient has METHYLMALONIC ACIDEMIA.

References

Gimsing, P., and Nexo, E. The forms of cobalamin in biological materials. Hall, C. A. (Ed.). *The Cobalamins*. Edinburgh: Churchill Livingstone, 1983, Chap. 1, p. 7.

Zittoun, J., and Marquet, J. Inherited disorders of cobalamin metabolism. J. Zittoun and B. A. Cooper (Eds.). *Folates and Cobalamins*. Berlin: Springer-Verlag, 1989, Chap. 18, p. 219.

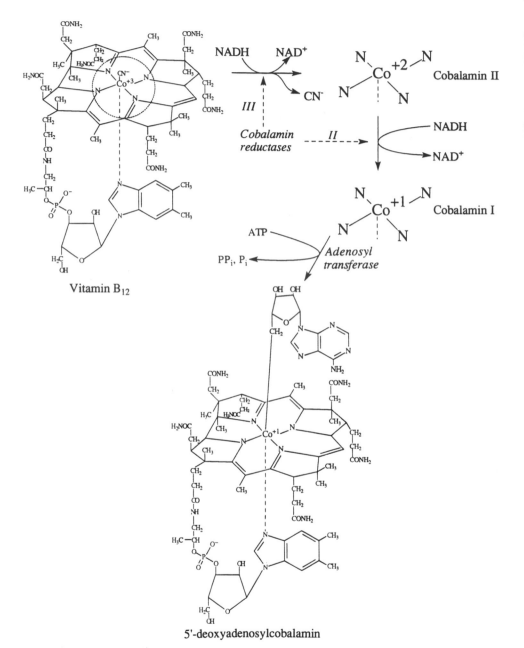

Vitamin B$_{12}$

5'-deoxyadenosylcobalamin

FIGURE A31-1. **Synthesis of deoxyadenosylcobalamin.** The dashed circle in the structure of vitamin B$_{12}$ represents the area that is expanded in the panels on the upper right, showing the reduction of the Co^{3+} to Co^{+1} by cobalamin reductases III and II.

Answer 32

a. Pernicious anemia is due to a deficiency in vitamin B_{12} (cobalamin). This could be dietary or due to lack of transport or uptake of cobalamin. The most common cause of pernicious anemia is lack of *intrinsic factor,* a protein that complexes with cobalamin in the intestine and allows it to be taken up by the intestine. However, both your patients have normal intrinsic factor and normal levels of cobalamin in their blood; hence we must eliminate poor diet or lack of intrinsic factor as causes of the problem. Therefore, the problem must be connected to transport, uptake, or metabolism of cobalamin further down the line. However, both your patients have very low levels of cobalamin in their liver cells, which restricts the possible defects to transport or uptake of cobalamin.

Cobalamin is not transported free in the blood, but complexed to a family of carrier proteins called *transcobalamins,* in which there are three members: transcobalamins I, II, and III, which appear to be related to each other and to intrinsic factor. Most of the uptake of cobalamin by tissues involves transcobalamin II. The transcobalamin II–cobalamin complex then binds to a receptor in the liver cells and is taken up. In the case of patient 1, his liver cells can take up radioactive cobalamin from a normal person's serum, but normal liver cells cannot take up cobalamin from your patient's serum. This suggests that the receptor is normal and that the transcobalamin II is abnormal. The situation is actually more complex because, although most dietary cobalamin is complexed immediately to transcobalamin II and then taken up by the tissues, the vast majority of the serum cobalamin is complexed to transcobalamin I, a protein whose actual function is unknown. This is the reason why your patient has normal levels of cobalamin in his serum.

b. In the case of patient 2, his liver cells cannot take up the radioactive cobalamin even from normal serum, which would contain normal transcobalamin II. Thus the problem with patient 2 must be the *receptor* for the transcobalamin II–cobalamin complex. This is further substantiated by the observation that patient 2's serum will allow radioactive cobalamin to be taken up by normal cells. The overall identification of the problems with your two patients is corroborated by the fact that patient 2's serum, which contains normal transcobalamin II, is able to support the uptake of radioactive cobalamin into patient 1's cells, which contain normal receptor.

References

Fenton, W. A., and Rosenberg, L. E. Inherited disorders of cobalamin transport and metabolism. C. R. Scriver, A. L. Beaudet, W. S. Sly, and D. Valle (Eds.). *The Metabolic Basis of Inherited Disease.* New York: McGraw-Hill, 1989, Vol. II, Chap. 82, p. 2065.

Johnston, J., Yang-Feng, T., and Berliner, N. "Genomic structure and mapping of the chromosomal gene for transcobalamin I (TCN1): comparison to human intrinsic factor." *Genomics* 12: 459, 1992.

Platica, O., Janeczko, R., Quadros, E. V., Regec, A., Romain, R., and Rothenberg, S. P. "The cDNA sequence and the deduced amino acid sequence of human transcobalamin II show homology with rat intrinsic factor and human transcobalamin I." *J. Biol. Chem.* 266: 7860, 1991.

Answer 33

a. The variety of acids that are elevated suggests a defect that has widespread effects. Your enzyme assays indicate that the enzymes which convert propionyl-CoA to methylmalonyl-CoA, pyruvate to oxaloacetate, and 3-methylcrotonyl-CoA to 3-methylglutaconyl-CoA are defective; these enzymes are, respectively, propionyl-CoA carboxylase, pyruvate carboxylase, and β-methylcrotonyl-CoA carboxylase. Excess propionyl-CoA can be converted into methylcitrate and 3-hydroxypropionate, while excess 3-methylcrotonyl CoA can be converted into 3-methylcrotonyl glycine. Thus defects in these enzyme could lead to the effects observed.

What do these enzymes have in common? All of them are carboxylases that use biotin as a coenzyme. Biotin is covalently attached to the carboxylases by the enzyme *holocarboxylase synthetase.* You find that biotin concentrations in your patient are normal. Therefore, the problem is not insufficient dietary biotin or poor uptake of biotin. The fact that radioactive biotin is not incorporated into proteins suggests that the holocarboxylase synthetase is defective. The holocarboxylase synthetase reaction is shown in Figure A33-1.

b. The cycle by which biotin is bound to and released from a carboxylase is shown in Figure A33-1.

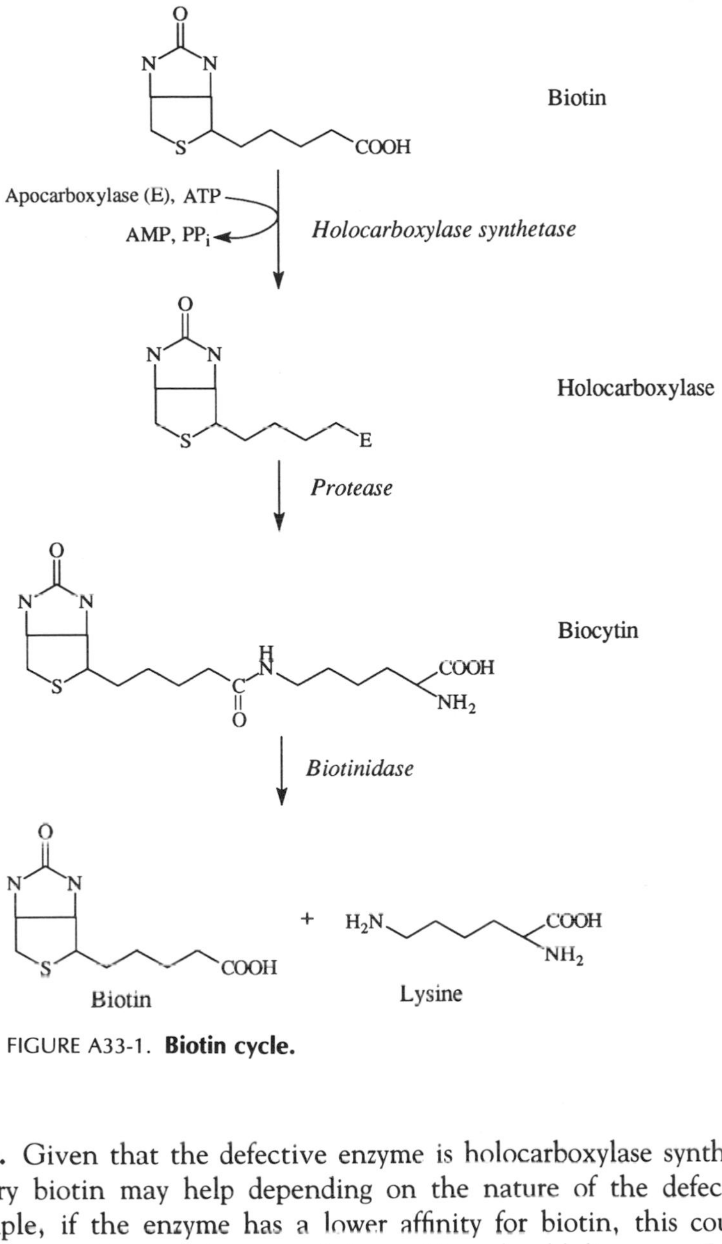

FIGURE A33-1. **Biotin cycle.**

c. Given that the defective enzyme is holocarboxylase synthetase, dietary biotin may help depending on the nature of the defect. For example, if the enzyme has a lower affinity for biotin, this could be overcome with excess biotin and the problem should disappear. By contrast, if the enzyme does not bind to biotin at all, increasing dietary biotin would not help. Also, the defect in the enzyme could be in the catalytic mechanism or in its binding to holocarboxylase or ATP; in these cases also, excess dietary biotin would have no effect. These latter defects would be extremely severe since processes such as gluconeogenesis would be inhibited.

Reference

Wolf, B., and Heard, G. S. Disorders of biotin metabolism. C. R. Scriver, A. L. Beaudet, W. S. Sly, and D. Valle (Eds.). *The Metabolic Basis of Inherited Disease.* New York: McGraw-Hill, 1989, Vol. II, Chap. 83, p. 2083.

CHAPTER 6

Minerals

Problem 34

This is a hypothetical problem. It is conceivable that someone could live for several months on an artificial diet entirely lacking the element selenium. Such a person might eventually develop symptoms of hypothyroidism. The iodine level in his diet would be normal, as would the iodine content of his thyroid. You would find that the circulating levels of thyroxine would be normal but that the levels of 3, 5, 3'-triiodothyronine would be very low.

    a. Name the defective enzyme and state what the enzyme does.

    b. Why would a deficiency in selenium affect this enzyme?

    c. What other enzyme contains selenium? How does selenium get incorporated into this enzyme?

Problem 35

Your patient is a 2-month-old boy with frequent vomiting, seizures, and psychomotor retardation. You do a liver biopsy and find that levels of sulfite (SO_3^{2-}) are very high. Xanthine oxidase activity in the isolated cells is very low. Analysis of his blood suggests that his diet is completely adequate.

a. What is wrong with your patient?

b. What is the structure of the defective substance, and how is it made?

c. Would you expect his aldehyde oxidase activity to be high or low? Why?

Problem 36

Your patient has hyperchloremic metabolic acidosis. He has low plasma HCO_3^-. Urinary levels of HCO_3^- are considerably higher than normal. You identify the problem as a manifestation of proximal renal tubular acidosis. The system by which the kidney reabsorbs HCO_3^- involves the following proteins: an apical membrane Na^+/H^+ antiporter, a basolateral membrane Na^+/K^+-ATPase, an apical membrane H^+-ATPase, a basolateral membrane $Na(HCO_3^-)_3$ symporter, and a luminal carbonic anhydrase. Describe the mechanisms by which the high urinary levels of HCO_3^- could be generated, assuming an isolated defect in one of the following:

a. The apical membrane Na^+/H^+ antiporter

b. The basolateral membrane Na^+/K^+-ATPase

c. The apical membrane of H^+-ATPase

Problem 37

Your patient is a very short 2-year-old child from a Bedouin tribe whose family history shows a great number of intermarriages within the tribe. She has skeletal deformities and bone pain. You would diagnose her symptoms as due to rickets except that her serum levels of $1\alpha,25$-dihydroxycholecalciferol are elevated. Her serum levels of phosphate are very low, and parathyroid hormone is low. Urinary concentrations of phosphate and calcium are high. Tests with oral calcium and phosphate show that calcium and phosphate are very readily absorbed through the intestine. Injection with parathyroid hormone causes an increase in cyclic AMP concentration in the urine. You find that oral calcium alone does not help your patient. Oral vitamin D does not help, nor do injections of $1\alpha,25$-dihydroxycholecalciferol. However, the symptoms virtually disappear when phosphate is introduced into the diet.

a. What is likely to be the defective protein in your patient?

b. How does this defect lead to rickets?

Problem 38

Your patient's lungs contain large amounts of a thick mucous secretion that makes breathing difficult and makes her susceptible to pneumonia and other pulmonary infections, which can be life-threatening. Her pancreatic digestive enzymes are low, so that she has fatty stools and is a slow grower. When she sweats a lot, crystals of sodium chloride appear on her skin. The concentration of chloride ion in her lung secretions is abnormally low. You find that there is a protein in the airway epithelium which is altered in your patient. Using the appropriate plasmid, you transfect the gene for either the altered or the normal protein into cultured epithelial cells from your patient and from a normal person. You measure chloride transport and obtain the results shown in Table P38-1.

You compare the sequences of the altered and the normal protein. You find that phenylalanine in position 508 of the normal protein is deleted in your patient's protein. The sequence in this region in the normal person is likely to form a β sheet.

Using an antibody to the protein, you do immunofluorescence and find that your patient's protein is located near the nucleus and not on the membrane, whereas a normal person would have the protein located in many parts of the cell, including the membrane. You also observe that the protein from a normal person is glycosylated, whereas your patient's protein is not.

You purify the altered protein from your patient and then reconstitute it with phospholipids to make a liposome; you then measure chloride transport and find that it is normal.

You incubate your patient's protein and the equivalent protein from a normal person with the protein calnexin and find that they both bind equally well, but within a short time the calnexin releases the normal protein but not your patient's protein.

TABLE P38-1

Source of Epithelial Cells	Source of Transfected Protein	Chloride Transported (% of control)
Normal person	None	100
Your patient	None	5
Your patient	Your patient	10
Your patient	Normal person	100

a. What is the normal function of the protein that is altered in your patient?

b. Fill in the causative chain between the alteration in the protein and the symptoms. Be sure to explain all the experimental results described above. Feel free to speculate.

Problem 39

Your patient is a 5-year-old boy who has lost his baby teeth early. He appears to have rickets and took a long time in learning to walk. Serum levels of phosphoethanolamine, inorganic pyrophosphate, and pyridoxal-5'-phosphate are much higher than normal. Intracellular levels of pyridoxal-5'-phosphate are normal. You collect some blood and add to it radioactive pyrophosphate and measure the release of radioactive phosphate. You find that the release is much less than normal. You do a biopsy of the intestine, prepare a cell-free extract, and add radioactive pyrophosphate to the extract. Here you find that release of radioactive phosphate is normal.

a. Name the defective enzyme. Is it intracellular or extracellular?

b. How do you account for the observation that the enzyme reaction was normal in the intestine and subnormal in the blood?

c. Despite the increased extracellular levels of pyridoxal-5'-phosphate, how do you account for the fact that your patient does not exhibit vitamin B_6 toxicity?

Problem 40

Your patient is mentally retarded. Her bones appear abnormally dense on x-rays. CT scan reveals calcification in portions of her brain. You do a bone biopsy and purify the osteoclasts. You prepare a cell-free extract and add radioactive CO_2. You find that production of HCO_3^- is abnormally low.

a. Name the defective enzyme and state what it does.

b. How could this defect account for the extradense bone?

Answer 34

a. Thyroxine levels are normal, implying that there is no problem in synthesizing the thyroid hormones. The low levels of 3,5,3'-triiodothyronine (T_3) suggest that the defective enzyme is the one that converts thyroxine to T_3. We have two enzymes capable of carrying out this reaction: type I and type II iodothyronine 5'-deiodinase. Type I contains selenium, whereas type II does not. The type I enzyme is found in the liver and the kidney and is thought to play a major role in determining levels of T_3. The type II enzyme is found in the pituitary and in brown adipose tissue and is thought to play a role in local conversion of thyroxine to T_3. For these reasons it is likely that the defective enzyme is *type I iodothyronine 5'-deiodinase*, which catalyzes the reaction shown in Figure A34-1.

Since T_3 is more active than thyroxine, the person with the defective enzyme would be likely to have symptoms of hypothyroidism.

b. Type I iodothyronine 5'-deiodinase contains the amino acid selenocysteine, which is important in the catalytic activity.

c. Selenium is part of glutathione peroxidase, which catalyzes this reaction:

$$2GSH + H_2O_2 \rightarrow GSSG + 2H_2O$$

Selenium is an essential trace element in our diet. Although selenium deficiency is very rare, it occurs in certain areas of rural China, where

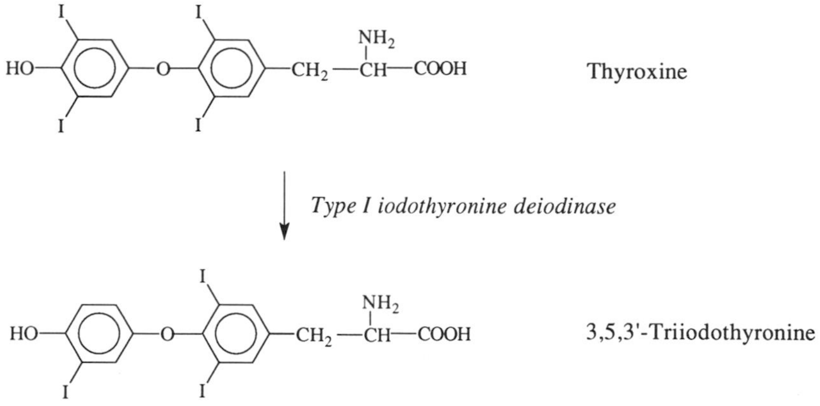

FIGURE A34-1. **Iodothyronine 5'-deiodinase reaction.**

it is called Keshan disease; it occurs among children of peasants who grow all their own food in selenium-poor soil. One of the symptoms is cardiomyopathy.

Selenium is part of the residue *selenocysteine*. Notice the similarity to cysteine and serine (Figure A34-2). Obviously, selenocysteine is not one of the 20 fundamental amino acids incorporated into proteins by the normal protein biosynthetic process. However, synthesis of selenocysteine is not done by posttranslational modification, but rather, by what could be considered *cotranslational modification*. The process is shown in Figure A34-3. First, an amino acyl tRNA synthetase adds serine to a special tRNA, which has a variety of unique structural features. Second, the enzyme *selenocysteine synthase* replaces the oxygen of serine with a selenium atom to make selenocysteinyl-tRNA.

When deiodinase is made on the ribosome, the tRNA^{Sec} recognizes a UGA codon in the main reading frame and inserts selenocysteine at this position, which is 126 in the amino acid sequence. In short, free selenocysteine does not bind to tRNA and does not get incorporated into proteins.

Why is this UGA not read as a STOP codon? There is a long untranslated region at the 3' end of the mRNA molecule. The open reading frame on the mRNA is from nucleotides 7 to 780; the 3'-untranslated region goes from 781 to 2106. There is a segment in this region between nucleotides 1440 and 1615 which controls how the UGA codon (at nucleotides 382 to 384) is read. If the UGA codon is mutated to UGU, which codes for cysteine, the enzyme is made with cysteine instead of selenocysteine at position 126; it is fully active but with a 10-fold higher K_m value for 3,5,3'-triiodothyronine. Removal of this segment in the 3'-untranslated region has no effect on the activity of the mutant enzyme. With the normal enzyme that has the UGA codon, however, removal of this segment prevents synthesis of active enzyme, presumably

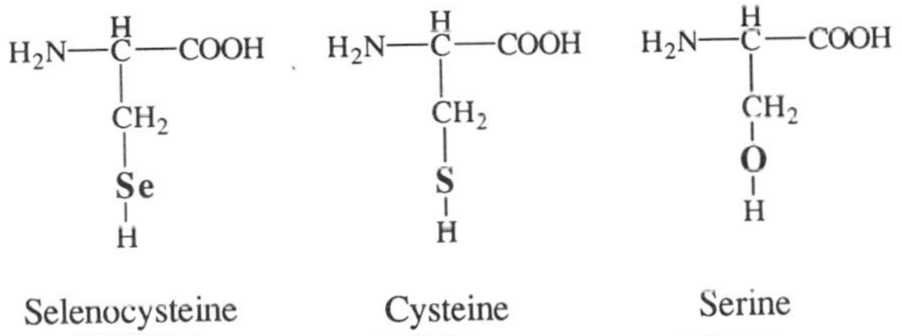

FIGURE A34-2. **Structures of selenocysteine, cysteine, and serine.**

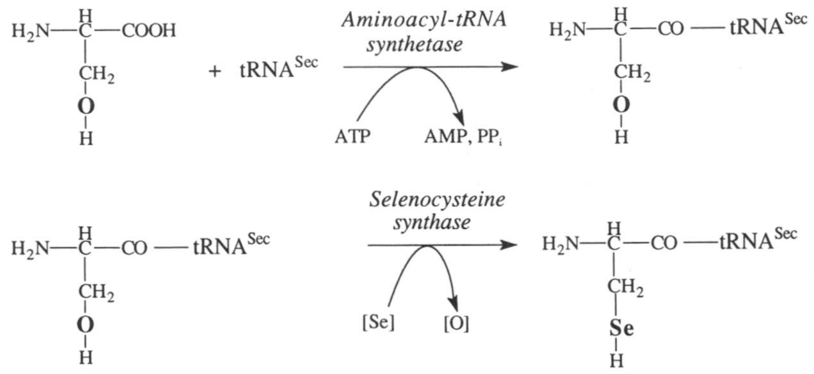

FIGURE A34-3. **Incorporation of selenium into proteins.**

by causing the ribosome to read UGA as a STOP codon rather than as selenocysteine. This segment of the mRNA therefore controls how the UGA codon is read. If it is present, the UGA codes for selenocysteine. Interestingly, an analogous segment is present in the 3′ untranslated region of the mRNA for glutathione peroxidase and two such segments are present in the mRNA for selenoprotein P, the only other known selenium-containing protein in mammals; selenoprotein P contains about 8 to 10 UGA codons, each of which is read as selenocysteine. In each case the segment can be predicted to form a stem loop structure. Removal of the eight residues likely to form the loop completely inhibits expression of the deiodinase or the peroxidase. It appears that there is a unique factor, perhaps an elongation factor, which recognizes the secondary structure of the mRNA, specifically the loop region. It is postulated that a complex of this factor with the stem-loop region can somehow interact with the UGA codon to ensure that selenocysteinyl-tRNA binds at that position.

Is there any way for free selenocysteine to become incorporated into proteins directly? The answer is no. In fact, there is an enzyme, *selenocysteine lyase,* which degrades selenocysteine into alanine and hydrogen selenide (H_2Se).

References

Berry, M. J., Banu, L., Chen, Y., Mandel, S. J., Kieffer, J. D., Harney, J. W., and Larsen, P. R. Recognition of UGA as a selenocysteine codon in type I deiodinase requires sequences in the 3′ untranslated region. *Nature* 353: 273, 1991.

Berry, M. J., Banu, L., Harney, J. W., and Larsen, P. R. Functional characterization of the eukaryotic SECIS elements which direct selenocysteine insertion at UGA codons. *EMBO J.* 12: 3315, 1993.

Berry, M. J., Banu, L., and Larsen, P. R. Type I iodothyronine deiodinase is a selenocysteine-containing enzyme. *Nature* 349: 438, 1991.

Berry, M. J., and Larsen, P. R. Molecular cloning of the selenocysteine-containing enzyme type I iodothyronine deiodinase. *Am. J. Clin. Nutr. Suppl.* 57: 249S, 1993.

Daher, R., and Van Lente, F. Characterization of selenocysteine lyase in human tissues and its relationship to tissue selenium concentrations. *J. Trace Elem. Electrolytes Health Dis.* 6: 189, 1992.

Hill, K. E., Lloyd, R. S., and Burk, R. F. Conserved nucleotide sequences in the open reading frame and 3' untranslated region of selenoprotein P mRNA. *Proc. Natl. Acad. Sci. USA* 90: 537, 1993.

Litov, R. E., and Combs, G. F. Selenium in pediatric nutrition. *Pediatrics* 87: 339, 1991.

Liu, S. Y., and Wang, F. Damage to hepatic thyroxine 5'-deiodination induced by pathogenic factors of Keshan disease and the preventive effects of selenium and vitamin E. *Biomed. Environ. Sci.* 4: 359, 1991.

Shen, Q., Chu, F.-F., and Newburger, P. E. Sequences in the 3'-untranslated region of the human glutathione cellular peroxidase gene are necessary and sufficient for selenocysteine incorporation at the UGA codon. *J. Biol. Chem.* 268: 11463, 1993.

Sturchler, C., Westhof, E., Carbon, P., and Krol, A. Unique secondary and tertiary structural features of the eukaryotic selenocysteine tRNA[Sec]. *Nucleic Acids Res.* 21: 1073, 1993.

Answer 35

a. If sulfite (SO_3^{2-}) is high, the metabolism of sulfite must be blocked. The major route for metabolism of sulfite is catalyzed by *sulfite oxidase,* which converts sulfite to sulfate (SO_4^{2-}). Sulfite oxidase, is therefore, likely to be defective in your patient. Your patient is also defective in xanthine oxidase. These two enzymes are not in related pathways, so it is unlikely that a block in the activity of one would affect the other. It appears, therefore, that the missing factor must be something that the two enzymes have in common. The most logical candidate is the metal ion molybdenum, which both enzymes require. Your patient's diet is normal, so it is not likely that he is suffering from molybdenum deficiency. However, molybdenum does not operate by itself in proteins, but is complexed with a pterin derivative called *molybdenum cofactor,* also known as molybdopterin. This must therefore be the defective substance (Figure A35-1).

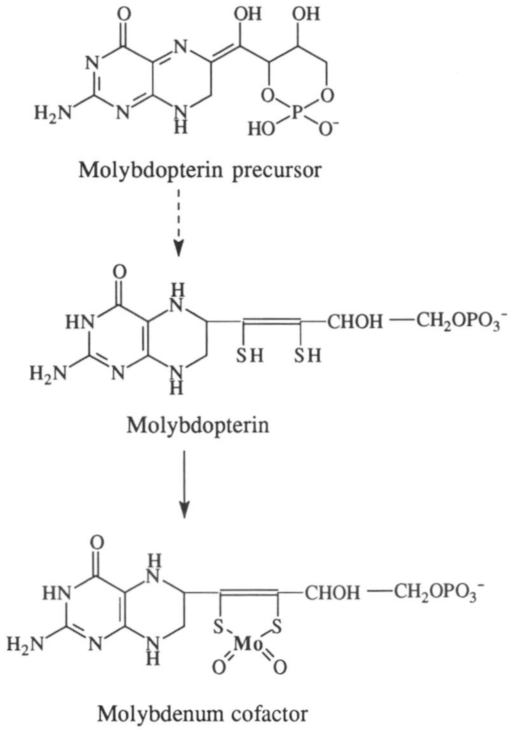

FIGURE A35-1. **Possible biosynthesis of molybdopterin.**

b. The pathway of biosynthesis of molybdopterin in humans has not yet been elucidated; in the bacterium *Escherichia coli*, however, molybdopterin is made from the *molybdopterin precursor* (Figure A35-1). One reason for the difficulty in elucidating the pathway is the instability of molybdopterin, whose vicinal sulfhydryls are very reactive. Interestingly, Archaebacteria also have a molybdenum cofactor, but the molybdenum is replaced by a tungsten atom.

c. You would expect aldehyde oxidase activity to be low because aldehyde oxidase also requires molybdenum.

References

Gardlik, S., and Rajagopalan, K. V. The state of reduction of molybdopterin in xanthine oxidase and sulfite oxidase. *J. Biol. Chem.* 265: 13047, 1990.

Johnson, J. L., Rajagopalan, K. V., Mukund, S., and Adams, M. W. W. Identification of molybdopterin as the organic component of the tungsten cofactor in four enzymes from hyperthermophilic Archaea. *J. Biol. Chem.* 268: 4848, 1993.

Johnson, J. L., and Wadman, S. K. Molybdenum cofactor deficiency. C. R. Scriver, A. L. Beaudet, W. S. Sly, and D. Valle (Eds.). *The Metabolic Basis of Inherited Disease.* New York: McGraw-Hill, 1989, Vol. I, Chap. 56, p. 1463.

Pitterle, D. M., Johnson, J. L., and Rajagopalan, K. V. In vitro synthesis of molybdopterin from precursor Z using purified converting factor: role of protein-bound sulfur in formation of the dithiolene. *J. Biol. Chem.* 268: 13506, 1993.

Pitterle, D. M., and Rajagopalan, K. V. The biosynthesis of molybdopterin in *Escherichia coli*: purification and characterization of the converting factor. *J. Biol. Chem.* 268: 13499, 1993.

Wuebbens, M. M., and Rajagopalan, K. V. Structural characterization of a molybdopterin precursor. *J. Biol. Chem.* 268: 13493, 1993.

Answer 36

a. The antiporter pumps H^+ out of the cell in exchange for sodium. The driving force is the sodium gradient. The H^+ reacts with HCO_3^- to form H_2CO_3, which reacts with carbonic anhydrase to form CO_2 and H_2O. CO_2 reabsorbs freely. A defect in the antiporter would lead to less H^+ in the lumen and less H_2CO_3 formed; hence there would be high HCO_3^-. In other words, in the equation

$$HCO_3^- + H^+ \rightarrow H_2CO_3$$

decreasing the H^+ concentration in the lumen would lead to less H_2CO_3 being made.

b. The basolateral membrane Na/K-ATPase pumps Na^+ out of the cell against a gradient. It requires energy. Creation of this gradient drives H^+ excretion. A defect in this pump would lower the H^+ concentration in the lumen.

c. The apical membrane H^+-ATPase pumps H^+ out of the cell into the lumen. The H^+ reacts with HCO_3^- to form H_2CO_3, which reacts with carbonic anhydrase to form CO_2 and H_2O. CO_2 reabsorbs freely. A defect in apical membrane H^+ ATPase would lead to less H^+ in the lumen and less H_2CO_3 formed; hence there would be high HCO_3^-.

Reference

DuBose, T. D., and Alpern, R. J. Renal tubular acidosis. C. R. Scriver, A. L. Beaudet, W. S. Sly, and D. Valle (Eds.). *The Metabolic Basis of Inherited Disease.* New York: McGraw-Hill, 1989, Vol. II, Chap. 103, p. 2539.

Answer 37

a. Having symptoms like those of rickets suggests a major problem in the metabolism of bone: either not enough calcium and phosphate are being deposited in the bone or too much calcium and phosphate are being dissolved from the bone. The fact that levels of $1\alpha,25$-dihydroxycholecalciferol are high eliminates the possibility that he has a vitamin D deficiency, a common cause of rickets; vitamin D is a precursor of $1\alpha,25$-dihydroxycholecalciferol. Parathyroid hormone levels are low; if they were high, this might help to explain the symptoms, since high concentrations of parathyroid hormone can remove calcium phosphate from bone. Since this is not the case, however, parathyroid hormone levels cannot be the culprit here. Thus the two major regulators of bone metabolism seem to be functioning properly.

Let us examine the uptake and transport of calcium and phosphate, the constituents of bone. Uptake of calcium and phosphate is normal. Urinary concentrations of calcium and phosphate are high, but phosphate levels in the blood are low. Clearly, there is no problem in taking either calcium or phosphate up in the intestine. The most intriguing fact is that phosphate is low in the blood and high in the urine. If normal amounts of phosphate are consumed and phosphate is not being deposited in the bone, blood phosphate should be high. The fact that it is high in the urine and low in the blood means that phosphate reabsorption in the kidney is defective. Hence the defect is likely to lie in the *renal phosphate transporter*.

b. Bone is a mineral: it is calcium phosphate with the approximate composition $Ca_{10}(PO_4)_6(OH)_2$. Defects in the metabolism of either calcium or phosphate could in principle lead to poor mineralization of bone and therefore to symptoms of rickets. In this case the problem is with renal phosphate reabsorption in the kidney. With low circulating levels of phosphate, mineralization is inhibited regardless of the amount of calcium present in the diet. Since much of the calcium that would normally be deposited in the bone is unable to do so, the calcium concentrations in the urine are high. The problem can be solved by increasing the phosphate in the diet of the child. The higher phosphate can compensate for the poorly functioning phosphate transporter in the kidney.

Reference

Rasmussen, H., and Tenenhouse, H. S. Hypophosphatemias. C. R. Scriver, A. L. Beaudet, W. S. Sly, and D. Valle (Eds.). *The Metabolic Basis of Inherited Disease.* New York: McGraw-Hill, 1989, Vol. II, Chap. 105, p. 2581.

Answer 38

a. Your patient has a defect of chloride transport that can be corrected by transfection of a certain protein from a normal person. The fact that transfecting her own protein does not solve the problem indicates that the act of transfection per se does not in some way permit chloride transport to happen. Clearly, the defective protein is involved in transport of chloride ion. In the sweat glands, for example, there is a mechanism by which both sodium and chloride are transported together out of the lumen across the epithelium. If this is defective, both sodium and chloride accumulate in the sweat gland and cause deposition of salt crystals in the skin after the sweat evaporates. In the airways of a normal person, the secretion of chloride out of the epithelial cells into the lumen has the effect of hydrating the mucus secreted into the lumen and permitting its normal clearance. If chloride ion transport is inhibited, the mucus accumulates and becomes thick. The clogged airways are ideal environments for growth of *Pseudomonas* and *Staphylococcus,* which cause lung infections that are difficult to treat and are often ultimately fatal. The protein that is altered in your patient is known as the *cystic fibrosis transmembrane conductance regulator* (CFTR).

b. Your experiments indicate that your patient's protein is functional because when it is in a liposome, it is able to conduct chloride ion normally. The problem appears to be with the localization or processing. In a normal person, the protein gets to the membrane, but not in your patient. In a normal person, the protein gets glycosylated but not in your patient. This cannot be from loss of a glycosylation site, since phenylalanine is not such a site. It does seem that there is a problem processing your protein. The finding with calnexin is most revealing. Calnexin is a *chaperonin;* these are a family of proteins that help other proteins fold properly. In general, a chaperonin binds to a protein, helps it to fold, and then releases it. The fact that calnexin has trouble releasing your patient's protein suggests that the mutation in the protein, although not affecting its function, could affect its interaction with calnexin in such a way that the protein does not get processed correctly and never reaches its destination. Perhaps the altered protein cannot rearrange its conformation so as to bury its hydrophobic areas, and that may keep it trapped inside the chaperonin.

   Why would the deletion of phenylalanine 508 have this effect? It is difficult to say, except that position 508 is speculated to be in a β sheet. These are structures in which the amino acid side chains alternate in the direction in which they point out from the polypeptide backbone. If there is a deletion in the sheet, there are two possibilities. One is that the sheet will disappear and be replaced by another type of structure.

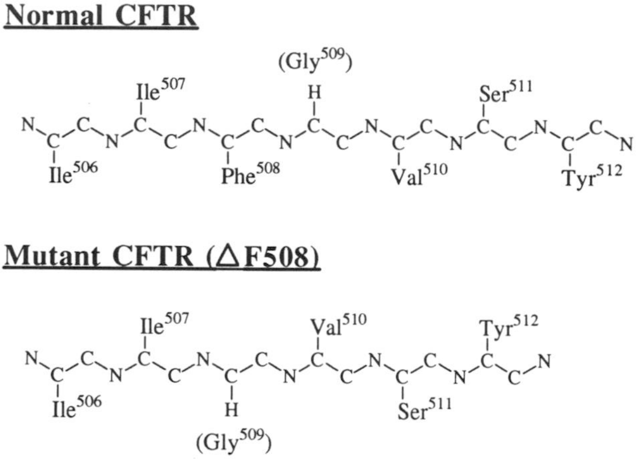

FIGURE A38-1. **Effect of deletion of Phe^{508} on β-sheet structure. In this figure we are looking at the β sheet from the side; the hydrogen bonds maintaining the structure are perpendicular to the plane of the figure and are not shown. The figure shows the orientation of the side chains. Notice how in normal CFTR, the hydrophobic side chains of Ile^{506}, Phe^{508}, Val^{510}, and Tyr^{512} are all pointing in the same direction. When Phe^{508} is deleted, however, the polar side chain of Ser^{511} is now pointing in that direction and the nonpolar side chains of Val^{510} and Tyr^{512} are in a region that may have been polar in normal CFTR. Also a moderately bulky Val^{510} has its side chain where normal CFTR has a glycine (with no side chain).**

This could easily have large effects on the interaction of the protein with other proteins. A second possibility is that the sheet remains intact, but being one amino acid shorter, the directions of the side chains will now be rearranged as shown in Figure A38-1. This could also have substantial effects on the conformation of the whole protein and may affect its interaction with calnexin.

Your patient has CYSTIC FIBROSIS.

References

Boat, T. F., Welsh, M. J., and Beaudet, A. L. Cystic fibrosis. C. R. Scriver, A. L. Beaudet, W. S. Sly, and D. Valle (Eds.). *The Metabolic Basis of Inherited Disease.* New York: McGraw-Hill, 1989, Vol. II, Chap. 108, p. 2649.

Cheng, S. H., Gregory, R. J., Marshal, L. J., Paul, S., Souza, D. W., White, G. A., O'Riordan, C. R., and Smith, A. E. Defective intracellular transport and processing of CFTR is the molecular basis of most cystic fibrosis. *Cell* 63: 827, 1990.

Dalemans, W., Barbry, P., Champigny, G., Jallat, S., Dott, K., Dreyer, D., Crystal, R. G., Pavirani, A., Lecocq, J.-P., and Lazdunski, M. Altered chloride ion channel kinetics associated with the ΔF508 cystic fibrosis mutation. *Nature* 354: 526, 1991.

Gregory, R. J., Rich, D. P., Cheng, S. H., Souza, D. W., Paul, S., Manavalan, P., Anderson, M. P., Welsh, M. J., and Smith, A. E. Maturation and function of cystic fibrosis transmembrane conductance regulator variants bearing mutations in putative nucleotide-binding domains 1 and 2. *Mol. Cell. Biol.* 11: 3886, 1991.

Kerem, E., Corey, M., Kerem, B., Rommens, J., Markiewicz, D., Levison, H., Tsui, L.-C., and Durie, P. The relation between genotype and phenotype in cystic fibrosis: analysis of the most common mutation (ΔF_{508}). *New Engl. J. Med.* 323: 1517, 1990.

Pind, S., Riordan, J. R., and Williams, D. B. Participation of the ER chaperone calnexin (p88, IP90) in the biogenesis of CFTR. *J. Biol. Chem.* 269, 1994, in press.

Answer 39

a. There is clearly a difference in the conversion of pyrophosphate to phosphate, which occurs by the reaction

$$H_2P_2O_7^{2-} + H_2O \rightarrow 2H_2PO_4^-$$

The enzyme that carries out this reaction is *alkaline phosphatase*. This enzyme also removes phosphate groups from phosphoethanolamine and pyridoxal-5'-phosphate. The fact that the latter two compounds, as well as pyrophosphate, are high indicates that alkaline phosphatase is defective. Since pyridoxal-5'-phosphate levels inside the cells are normal, one concludes that alkaline phosphatase is an *extracellular* enzyme.

b. Alkaline phosphatase occurs as three isozymes. One isozyme is found largely in the intestine, one in the placenta, and the third is ubiquitous, although found largely in bone, liver, and kidney. It is possible that the intestinal isozyme may have both a fetal and an adult form. The precise function of alkaline phosphatase is not clear. It is possible that the intestinal and placental isozymes are involved in phosphate transport. The third isozyme, which is the form that is found in bone, may play a major role in mineralization, by binding calcium, destroying inhibitors of mineralization (such as pyrophosphate), or simply raising the local phosphate concentration. The reason that alkaline phosphatase activity was low in the blood and normal in the intestine is that the intestinal isozyme of alkaline phosphatase is normal. The defect in your patient involves the third isozyme of alkaline phosphatase, the isozyme which is found in many tissues including the serum and in bone.

c. Pyridoxal-5′-phosphate was normal *inside* the cells, which is where it counts. The source of pyridoxal-5′-phosphate is Vitamin B_6, a mixture of pyridoxol, pyridoxal and pyridoxamine. These compounds are converted to pyridoxal-5′-phosphate inside cells by a series of reactions that includes a kinase-catalyzed phosphorylation. The pyridoxal-5′-phosphate in the blood does not enter cells. The excess pyridoxal-5′-phosphate in the blood does not cause any problems.

Your patient has HYPOPHOSPHATASIA.

Reference

Whyte, M. P. Hypophosphatasia. C. R. Scriver, A. L. Beaudet, W. S. Sly, and D. Valle (Eds.). *The Metabolic Basis of Inherited Disease.* New York: McGraw-Hill, 1989, Vol. II, Chap. 116, p. 2843.

Answer 40

a. The defective enzyme must be involved in the conversion of CO_2 to HCO_3^-. This enzyme is *carbonic anhydrase,* which catalyzes the following reaction:

$$CO_2 + H_2O \leftrightarrow H_2CO_3$$

The H_2CO_3 thus produced immediately ionizes spontaneously:

$$H_2CO_3 \leftrightarrow H^+ + HCO_3^-$$

About six isozymes of carbonic anhydrase are likely to exist in humans. Of these, type IV is found in the lung and the kidney and is membrane-bound so that it is not likely to be found in a cell-free extract, even if it were to occur in the osteoclasts. Type V is found in liver mitochondria and would probably be pelleted with the mitochondria in preparation of a cell-free extract. Type VI is found in saliva and is therefore secreted and again not likely to be found in a cell-free extract from osteoclasts. Types I, II, and III are soluble and reasonable candidates to occur in cell-free extracts. Of these, type I generally occurs in erythrocytes and type III in skeletal muscle. Type II, by contrast, is very widespread and is therefore the most likely one to occur in osteoclasts. Thus the defective enzyme is probably *carbonic anhydrase II*.

b. Resorption of bone plays an important role in bone metabolism. For resorption to occur, the osteoclasts have to maintain an acidic pH outside the cells. This appears to be the job of an ATPase which pumps H^+ out across the cell membrane, thereby maintaining an extracellular pH of about 4.5. This generates H^+ by splitting H_2O to H^+ and OH^-. Presumably the OH^- remains inside the osteoclast. Carbonic anhydrase II, inside the osteoclast, causes regeneration of H^+. This H^+ then reacts with the OH^- to form H_2O. Without the carbonic anhydrase reaction, the OH^- levels in the osteoclast would build up to where the ATPase would not be pumping H^+ out of the cell.

Your patient has CARBONIC ANHYDRASE II DEFICIENCY SYNDROME, also known as GUIBAUD–VAINSEL SYNDROME.

Reference
Sly, W. S. The carbonic anhydrase II deficiency syndrome: osteopetrosis with renal tubular acidosis and cerebral calcification. C. R. Scriver, A. L. Beaudet, W. S. Sly, and D. Valle (Eds.). *The Metabolic Basis of Inherited Disease.* New York: McGraw-Hill, 1989, Vol. II, Chap. 117, p. 2857.

CHAPTER 7

Oxygen

Problem 41

Your patient has been relatively symptom-free except for a slightly high frequency of mouth sores. At one point you apply a dilute solution of hydrogen peroxide to the mouth sores and you notice that the adjacent tissue turns black instead of remaining colorless and bubbling. You draw some blood from your patient and isolate the erythrocytes. When you add hydrogen peroxide you get no bubbling; in contrast, with erythrocytes from a normal person, you would see bubbling. Analysis of the urine shows five times the normal concentration of bilirubin and coproporphyrin. There is no evidence of increased breakdown of erythrocytes or of liver dysfunction.

You isolate and sequence the gene coding for this enzyme and find the following sequence, compared to the sequence of the same gene from a normal person (exon sequences are underlined):

Your patient:	5'-TTGGTAGATAATA-3'
Normal person:	5'-TTGGTAGGTAATA-3'

a. Name the enzyme whose activity is decreased.

b. What is in the bubbles?

c. Explain how the observed change in the sequence could cause the disease. Speculate as to the cause of the increased bilirubin excretion, as well.

Answer 41

a. Your patient must have a defect in an enzyme that turns H_2O_2 into a substance that bubbles—that is, a gas. Our bodies have two pathways for getting rid of H_2O_2. One, catalyzed by a variety of peroxidases, turns H_2O_2 into water and an oxidized substrate. The other, catalyzed by *catalase*, turns H_2O_2 into water and O_2, which is a gas:

$$2H_2O_2 \rightarrow 2H_2O + O_2$$

Your patient must therefore be defective in catalase.

b. The bubbles must be made of O_2, which is the gas produced by the catalase reaction.

c. The increased level of bilirubin is a clue here. Unless we assume that there is an additional liver problem, the increased bilirubin level is likely to be due to increase in the degradation of heme-containing proteins. Often, that is a sign of hemolysis, the breakdown of erythrocytes and subsequent degradation of hemoglobin, but other heme-containing proteins could also be sources of heme. Catalase contains heme; increased degradation would increase bilirubin. Hence the defect might involve increased degradation of catalase.

Now, why do we have increased degradation of catalase? The observed base change is in an intron, not in an exon. The mutation is five residues away from an exon. Probably, the mutation leads to an error when the mRNA is spliced. The abnormal catalase thus produced may be very susceptible to degradation.

Your patient has ACATALASEMIA.

References

Eaton, J. W. Acatalasemia. C. R. Scriver, A. L. Beaudet, W. S. Sly, and D. Valle (Eds.). *The Metabolic Basis of Inherited Disease.* New York: McGraw-Hill, 1989, Vol. II, Chap. 60, p. 1551.

Kishimoto, Y., Murakami, Y., Hayashi, K., Takahara, S., Sugimura, T., and Sekiya, T. Detection of a common mutation of the catalase gene in Japanese acatalasemic patients. *Hum. Genet.* 88. 487, 1992.

Ogata, M., Acatalasemia. *Hum. Genet.* 86: 331, 1991.

Wen, J.-K., Osumi, T., Hashimoto, T., and Ogata, M. Molecular analysis of human acatalasemia: identification of a splicing mutation. *J. Mol. Biol.* 211: 383, 1990.

CHAPTER 8

Hormones

Problem 42

Your patient has a goiter and is developmentally delayed. Her circulating levels of thyroxine and triiodothyronine are very low. Your diagnosis is hypothyroidism. You observe that there is no problem with radioactive iodine being taken up by the thyroid. You do a thyroid biopsy and prepare a cell-free extract. You add radioactive iodide and find that virtually no radioactive thyroxine or triiodothyronine is made. In the presence of a high concentration of hematin, however, synthesis of thyroxine and triiodothyronine is normal. You find that thyroglobulin is normal.

a. Name the defective enzyme.

b. What is likely to be the precise defect in the enzyme?

Problem 43

Your patient has a goiter and is developmentally delayed. His circulating levels of thyroxine and triiodothyronine are low. Your diagnosis is hypothyroidism. You observe that there is no problem with radioactive iodine being taken up by the thyroid. You do a thyroid biopsy and prepare a cell-free extract. You add radioactive iodide and find that normal levels of radioactive monoiodotyrosine, diiodotyrosine, thyroxine, and triiodothyronine are made. You find that thyroglobulin is normal. You inject your patient with diiodotyrosine containing radioactive iodine and measure its excretion in the urine. You find that 15 times as much of the radioactive diiodotyrosine ends up in the urine as you would expect in a normal person. You put your patient on a high-iodine diet and his symptoms disappear.

a. Name the defective enzyme.

b. Why did the symptoms disappear when your patient was put on a diet with high levels of iodine?

Problem 44

Your patient has very low circulating levels of thyroxine. You find that injection of thyroid-stimulating hormone can produce normal levels of thyroxine. Injection of pyroglutamylhistidylprolinamide causes no production of thyroid-stimulating hormone. Your patient dies of causes unrelated to his disease. You recover the pituitary during autopsy. You add radioactive pyroglutamylhistidylprolinamide to the pituitary cells and find that the pyroglutamylhistidylprolinamide is not bound to the cells.

a. What is the likely defect in your patient?

b. Describe the roles of the hypothalamus and the pituitary in regulating the thyroid. How does thyroxine influence the secretion of thyroid-stimulating hormone?

Problem 45

Your patient is an infant with low sodium and high potassium levels in his blood. He is also dehydrated. He has in his blood elevated levels of 18-hydroxycorticosterone and very low levels of aldosterone.

Your patient has an altered enzyme. You purify the enzyme and incubate it with radioactive deoxycorticosterone. You find that production of radioactive 18-hydroxycorticosterone is significantly less than you would expect for a normal enzyme and that production of radioactive aldosterone is nil.

You look at the nucleotide sequence of the gene. You find the following result, compared to that for a normal person.

Codon number:	178	179	180	181	182	183
Your patient:	CAG	AAC	GCC	TGG	GGG	AGC
Normal person	CAG	AAC	GCC	CGG	GGG	AGC

a. Name the defective enzyme and write out the pathway by which progesterone is converted to aldosterone.

b. Identify the mutation and speculate as to the kinds of changes it would cause in the structure of the protein.

c. Given that your patient's enzyme in isolation has impaired synthesis of 18-hydroxycorticosterone, why does your patient have elevated levels of 18-hydroxycorticosterone?

Problem 46

Your patient was born with an abnormal penis in which the urethral opening is on the underside of the penis. He has low circulating levels of dehydroepiandrosterone, testosterone, and Δ^4-androstenedione. Other steroids are normal.

a. Name the defective enzyme.

b. Write out the pathway by which pregnenolone is converted to testosterone.

c. Why would you expect cyanide to inhibit this enzyme?

Problem 47

Your patient was an apparent hermaphrodite. He was a genetic male with female external genitalia and male internal genetic ducts. He had enlarged adrenals. His circulating levels of sodium were very low. Circulating levels of all steroids were very low, except for cholesterol. You prepare a cell-free extract from his adrenals and add radioactive cholesterol. You find that production of pregnenolone is very low. You find, however, that, if you add 20α-hydroxycholesterol, conversion into pregnenolone is normal.

a. Name the defective enzyme.

b. Why would you expect cyanide to exhibit this enzyme?

c. Describe the three steps of the reaction catalyzed by this enzyme.

Problem 48

Imagine that you have a patient with an accelerated basal metabolism and heartbeat. Her circulating levels of thyroxine, triiodothyronine, and thyroid-stimulating hormone are very high. As an experiment, you draw your patient's blood and add to it radioactive pyroglutamylhistidylprolinamide. After 10 minutes, you observe that the pyoglutamylhistidylproli namide is still present in the blood. In blood from a normal person, the pyroglutamylhistidylprolinamide would be gone in 10 minutes.

a. What is pyroglutamylhistidylprolinamide?

b. What is your patient's problem, and how does it lead to the elevated levels of thyroxine, triiodothyronine, and thyroid-stimulating hormone?

Problem 49

Your patient is an apparent hermaphrodite who is a genetic male with external female genitalia. Circulating levels of testosterone are normal for a male. You take a biopsy sample from genital skin fibroblasts and add [^{3}H]testosterone. You find that production of [^{3}H]dihydrotestosterone is 3% of that which you would find in a normal person. However, if you add much higher concentrations of [^{3}H]testosterone, you can get production of [^{3}H]dihydrotestosterone which is 20% of normal, but you cannot get higher than that no matter how much testosterone you add.

You are able to purify the defective enzyme and also clone and sequence its gene. The one change you observed in the gene is the following, at codon 34.

> Your patient: AGG
> Normal person: GGG

a. Name the defective enzyme and describe the reaction that it carries out.

b. How does this defect account for the phenotype? You find that your patient's internal genitalia (epididymis and vas deferens) are what you would expect for a male. Why is there a difference between the internal and external genitalia?

c. It turns out that normal persons have two enzymes that can carry out this reaction. Only one of these enzymes is defective in your patient. Why should your patient have any symptoms if he has one normal enzyme?

d. What exactly is the defect in your patient's enzyme?

Problem 50

A 15-year-old girl is brought to you by her mother because she has not had her period. You do a karyotype and find that she is really a boy, although her external anatomy is entirely that of a girl. It turns out that the patient's testes are in the abdomen. Circulating levels of testosterone are slightly higher than is normal for a male. The ratio of testosterone to dihydrotestosterone is normal. You culture some cells from the labia and add radioactive testosterone to them. You find that production of dihydrotestosterone is normal, but that unlike the normal case, the dihydrotestosterone does not localize to the nucleus.

You find that your patient has an altered gene. The partial sequence of your patient's gene and that of a normal person are as follows:

Codon number:	713	714	715	716	717	718	719	720	721	722
Your patient:	CAC	GTG	GTC	AAG	TGA	GCC	AAG	GCC	TTG	CCT
Normal person:	CAC	GTG	GTC	AAG	TGG	GCC	AAG	GCC	TTG	CCT

    a. Name the defective protein.

    b. How does this defect account for the phenotype?

    c. What is the nature of the defect in your patient's protein? Which of the functional properties of this protein would be most directly affected?

Problem 51

African pygmies have normal levels of human growth hormone and of insulin-like growth factor II. Prior to puberty the level of insulin-like growth factor I is normal, but its level does not rise during puberty. Unlike other people, African pygmies do not respond to injections of human growth hormone with an increase in insulin-like growth factor I.

a. Based on this information, what would you say is the role of the steroid sex hormones in mediating the effects of growth hormone?

b. What does insulin-like growth factor I do?

Problem 52

Your patient is of normal appearance. Phosphate levels in his blood are high and his calcium levels are low. His parathyroid hormone levels are high. You do a kidney biopsy and add parathyroid hormone to the cells. You find that cyclic AMP levels in the cell rise much less than you would expect in cells from a normal person. You do a thyroid biopsy and add thyroid-stimulating hormone to the thyroid cells; here the increase in cyclic AMP is normal. Then you do a liver biopsy and add glucagon; once again you find that cyclic AMP production is normal. You do one last experiment, in which you purify the membranes from your patient's kidney cells. You add to the membranes cholera toxin and radioactive ADP-ribose. You find that incorporation of radioactive label into a membrane protein is normal.

a. What is the defective protein likely to be?

b. If it had turned out that the cyclic AMP response was lower than normal in both the thyroid-stimulating hormone experiment and the glucagon experiment, what would you think that the defect in your patient is? Assume that the experiment with cholera toxins gives the same result.

Problem 53

Your patient appears to have rickets. Her rib cage is deformed; her teeth were late coming in and are poorly enamelized. She is 4 years old and unable to walk without support. Her muscles are very weak and her abdomen protrudes. She has no hair. Her blood tests show low calcium and high parathyroid hormone but normal levels of $1\alpha,25$-dihydroxycholecalciferol. If you treat this child with very high doses of $1\alpha,25$-dihydroxycholecalciferol, some improvement in the symptoms is noted. If you culture her fibroblasts and add small amounts of radioactive $1\alpha,25$-dihydroxycholecalciferol, very little binding to the cells results compared to what you would expect in a normal person. However, if you add very large amounts of $1\alpha,25$-dihydroxycholecalciferol, you get as much binding to the cells as you would get in a normal person.

a. Name the defective protein.

b. What exactly is wrong with the defective protein? Be as specific as you can.

Problem 54

Your patient was a man with an Irish surname born in the mountains of West Virginia. He just died after a 15-year struggle with amyloidosis. In the autopsy you discover aggregated protein in his nerves, heart, and thyroid. It was the gradually increasing amount of aggregated protein in his heart that was the cause of death. You identify the aggregated protein as transthyretin (also known as prealbumin). You did a liver biopsy on your patient shortly after his death and sequenced the gene, which was, in part, as follows:

Codon number:	59	60	61
Your patient:	ACA	GCT	GAG
Normal person:	ACA	ACT	GAG

a. How does your patient's transthyretin amino acid sequence differ from that of a normal person? How could this difference account for the deposition of this protein in aggregated form?

b. What is the normal function or functions of transthyretin?

Problem 55

Your patient has elevated levels of thyroxine in his system and has the symptoms of hyperthyroidism. You give him some ^{131}I and scan his thyroid. You find that there are certain regions in his thyroid where the radioactive iodine accumulates. The rest of the thyroid has less than a normal accumulation of ^{131}I. You do a biopsy and isolate a certain gene from the cells in the area that accumulate more ^{131}I than normal and from the cells in the area that accumulate less ^{131}I than normal. Let us call these cells "active" and "inactive," respectively. You sequence the genes and find that they differ. The differences are shown here together with the residue numbers in the protein for which this gene codes.

Residue number:	619	620	621	622	623	624	625	626	627	628	629	630
Active cells:	GAC	ACC	AAG	ATT	ATC	AAG	AGG	ATG	GCC	GTG	TTG	ATC
Inactive cells:	GAC	ACC	AAG	ATT	GCC	AAG	AGG	ATG	GCC	GTG	TTG	ATC

Further analysis of the sequence of the whole protein shows that it can be subdivided into regions which differ greatly in their relative contents of hydrophobic residues (Table P55-1). You also note that in region 1, the sequences Asn-X-Ser and Asn-X-Thr occur three times and two times, respectively.

TABLE P-55-1

Region	Residue Numbers	Hydrophobic Residues
1	1–415	198
2	416–440	22
3	441–450	3
4	451–473	18
5	474–494	10
6	495–516	13
7	517–537	11
8	538–560	20
9	561–581	12
10	582–605	19
11	606–625	7
12	626–648	18
13	649–661	7
14	662–681	16
15	682–764	35

You transfect both the gene from the active cells and the gene from the inactive cells into a cultured cell line. To these cells you then add a certain hormone and measure the production of cAMP by the cells. As a control you use cells that have been transfected only with the plasmid vector and not with one of these genes (Table P55-2).

a. What is the defective protein, and what is the hormone that you used in the experiment likely to be?

b. Which is mutated: the active or the inactive gene? How would the mutation lead to the observed phenotype? Why are both genes present?

c. Why are certain regions of the thyroid less active than normal?

TABLE P55-2

Transfection	Hormone	cAMP (arbitrary units)
Vector alone	No	2
	Yes	2
Active gene	No	16
	Yes	30
Inactive gene	No	6
	Yes	32

Problem 56

Your patient has hypertension. His serum has a high concentration of aldosterone and of 18-oxocortisol and 18-hydroxycortisol. If you treat him with glucocorticoids, his hypertension decreases and his levels of the foregoing three compounds go down to normal. You do an adrenal biopsy from your patient. You separate the cells from the zona glomerulosa and the zona fasciculata and do the following experiments, in which you compare the properties of these two types of cells from your patient and from a normal person. You add radioactive 18-hydroxycorticosterone and measure the production of radioactive aldosterone. The results are as follows:

	Zona Fasciculata	Zona Glomerulosa
Your patient:		
− ACTH:	20	20
+ ACTH:	100	100
Normal person:		
− ACTH:	0	20
+ ACTH:	0	100

You sequence certain regions of the genome and find that your patient has a normal gene for the enzyme you tested in the experiment and a normal gene for 11β-hydroxylase but that he has an additional chimeric gene consisting of the 5' regulatory region of 11β-hydroxylase and of the bulk of the gene coding for the enzyme whose activity you tested.

a. What is the enzyme whose activity you tested in the experiment?

b. How does the existence of the chimeric gene explain the results of the experiment?

c. Why does the condition respond to glucorticoid treatment?

Answer 42

a. The level of thyroid hormones is low. A deficiency in thyroid hormone synthesis could be due to many possibilities. The defect could be in the synthesis of thyroid-stimulating hormone or response to thyroid-stimulating hormone, or to a problem in the thyroid gland itself. The fact that the cell-free extract is unable to make thyroid hormone eliminates the first two of these possibilities. If the problem is in the thyroid, there are also several possibilities. Poor iodine uptake is clearly not the cause in this case. We are told that thyroglobulin appears to be normal. The fact that hematin (a derivative of heme) is able to correct the problem suggests that the problem is with *thyroperoxidase*, which is a heme-binding protein.

b. If the defect in thyroperoxidase can be corrected by adding a heme analog, the defect is likely to be in the binding of heme. In other words, your patient's thyroperoxidase may have a low affinity for heme.

Reference

Dumont, J. E., Vassart, G., and Refetoff, S. Thyroid disorders. C. R. Scriver, A. L. Beaudet, W. S. Sly, and D. Valle (Eds.). *The Metabolic Basis of Inherited Disease.* New York: McGraw-Hill, 1989, Vol. II, Chap. 73, p. 1843.

Answer 43

a. A defect in thyroid hormone synthesis could be due to a problem in the thyroid, the pituitary, or the hypothalamus. The fact that the symptoms disappear in the presence of excess dietary iodine suggests that the problem is located in the thyroid, which is the only organ that utilizes iodine. The lack of metabolism of diiodotyrosine suggests that the problem is in the enzyme that removes the iodine from diiodotyrosine: *iodotyrosine deiodinase* (Figure A43-1).

b. A person on a normal diet depends on the enzyme iodotyrosine deiodinase to recycle the iodine from the partly iodinated hormonal breakdown products and synthetic intermediates. If the enzyme is defective, much of this iodine will be excreted and not metabolized, and hence there will be a shortage of iodine. Excess iodine in the diet can compensate for this condition.

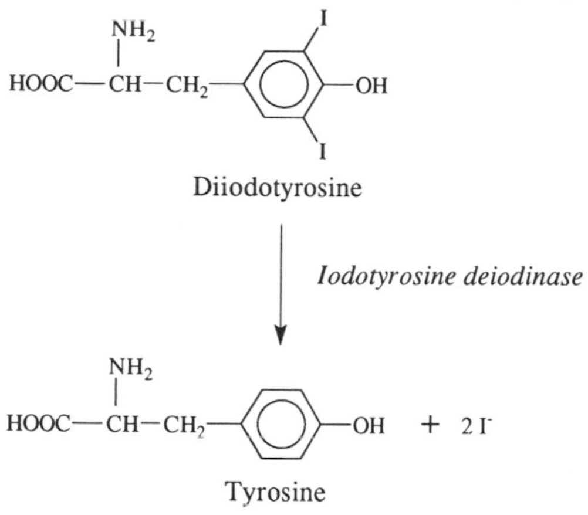

FIGURE A43-1. **Iodotyrosine deiodinase reaction.**

Reference

Dumont, J. E., Vassart, G., and Refetoff, S. Thyroid disorders. C. R. Scriver, A. L. Beaudet, W. S. Sly, and D. Valle (Eds.). *The Metabolic Basis of Inherited Disease.* New York: McGraw-Hill, 1989, Vol. II, Chap. 73, p. 1843.

Answer 44

a. Pyroglutamylhistidylprolinamide (Figure A44-1) is thyrotropin-releasing hormone, which is produced by the hypothalamus. Its target is the pituitary, which it induces to release thyroid-stimulating hormone (thyrotropin). If the pyroglutamylhistidylprolinamide is unable to bind to the pituitary, the defect is the lack of a receptor for thyrotropin-releasing hormone.

b. The hypothalamus produces thyrotropin-releasing hormone, which stimulates the pituitary to make thyroid-stimulating hormone, which in turn stimulates the thyroid to produce thyroxine and triiodothyronine. In the pituitary, thyroxine is converted to triiodothyronine which inhibits secretion of thyroid-stimulating hormone. Thus, the thyroid hormones feedback regulate their own synthesis.

Your patient has FAMILIAL PITUITARY HYPOTHYROIDISM.

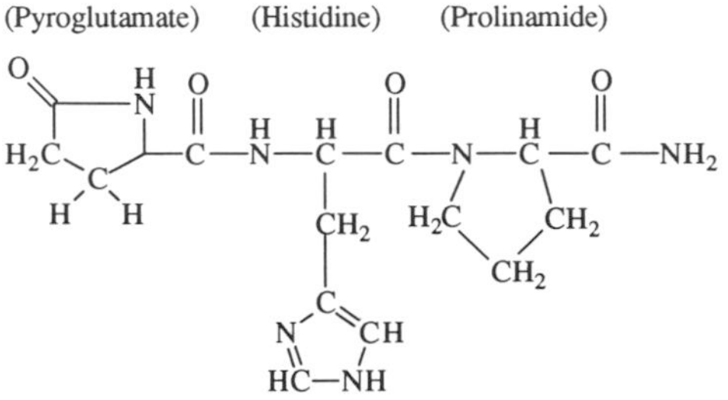

(Pyroglutamate)   (Histidine)   (Prolinamide)

Thyrotropin-releasing hormone (TRH)
(Pyroglutamylhistidylprolinamide)

FIGURE A44-1. **Structure of thyrotropin-releasing hormone.**

Reference

Dumont, J. E., Vassart, G., and Refetoff, S. Thyroid disorders. C. R. Scriver, A. L. Beaudet, W. S. Sly, and D. Valle (Eds.). *The Metabolic Basis of Inherited Disease.* New York: McGraw-Hill, 1989, Vol. II, Chap. 73, p. 1843.

Answer 45

a. Since aldosterone is low and 18-hydroxycorticosterone is high, the defective enzyme must be the one that converts 18-hydroxycorticosterone into aldosterone, namely *18-hydroxy dehydrogenase,* also known as *corticosterone methyl oxidase II* (Figure A45-1).

b. The mutation may be identified as follows:

Codon number:	178	179	180	181	182	183
Your patient:						
DNA:	CAG	AAC	GCC	TGG	GGG	AGC
RNA:	CAG	AAC	GCC	UGG	GGG	AGC
Protein:	Gln	Asn	Ala	Trp	Gly	Ser
Normal person:						
DNA:	CAG	AAC	GCC	CGG	GGG	AGC
RNA:	CAG	AAC	GCC	CGG	GGG	AGC
Protein:	Gln	Asn	Ala	Arg	Gly	Ser

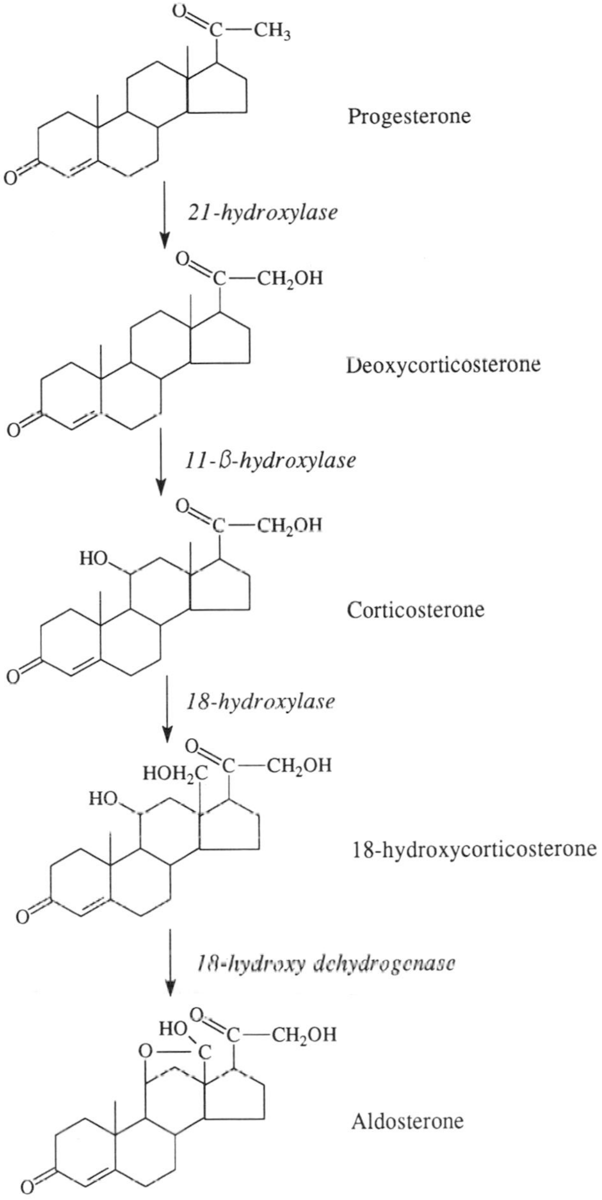

FIGURE A45-1. **Conversion of progesterone to aldosterone.** 18-Hydroxylase is also known as corticosterone methyl oxidase I.

Your patient has a mutation at position 181 in which an arginine is changed to a tryptophan. This is a drastic mutation. Arginine is a charged amino acid whose side chain is likely to be on the exterior of the protein, perhaps engaging in hydrogen or ionic bonds. The side chain could also be inside the protein if it is involved in an ionic bond. By contrast, tryptophan is uncharged and hydrophobic, very likely to be in the interior of a protein and not engaged in any but hydrophobic interactions. In short, this mutation could easily cause a drastic change in the structure of your patient's protein.

c. The question about why the purified enzyme has diminished ability to synthesize 18-hydroxycorticosterone whereas this compound is elevated in your patient is a complex one. To figure it out, you have to understand the nature of this enzyme. The enzyme is cytochrome P450cmo, which contains three activities: 11-hydroxylase, 18-hydroxylase, and 18-hydroxydehydrogenase (corticosterone methyl oxidase II). It turns out that there is another enzyme, almost an isozyme of this one, cytochrome P450cll, which has two activities: 11-β-hydroxylase and 18-hydroxylase. The mutation at position 181 in your patient's protein knocks out the 18-hydroxy dehydrogenase activity and diminishes the 18-hydroxylase activity, but the 18-hydroxylase activity in cytochrome P450cll compensates for the latter activity. Hence your patient uses cytochrome P450cll to make 18-hydroxycorticosterone, whose levels increase to higher-than-normal levels because it cannot be converted to aldosterone.

There is a further complexity. People with a defective enzyme also have a mutation in which position 386, which is normally a valine, is altered to alanine. This should be a relatively minor mutation. In reality, patients who have either just the mutation at position 181 or else the one at position 386 have no symptoms. To have symptoms, both mutations have to be present. Clearly, even though the mutation at position 386 is a relatively minor one, it must interact with the mutation at position 181 to produce a defective protein.

Your patient has ADRENAL HYPERPLASIA.

References

Globerman, H., Rösler, A., Theodor, R., New, M. I., and White, P. C. An inherited defect in aldosterone biosynthesis caused by a mutation in or near the gene for steroid 11-hydroxylase. *New Engl. J. Med.* 319: 1193, 1988.

Mitsuuchi, Y., Kawamoto, T., Naiki, Y., Miyahara, K., Toda, K., Kuribayashi, I., Orii, T., Yasuda, K., Miura, K., Nakao, K., Imura, H., Ulick, S., and Shizuta, Y. Congenitally defective aldosterone biosynthesis in humans: the involvement of point mutations of the P-450$_{C18}$ gene (CYP11B2) in CMO II deficient patients. *Biochem. Biophys. Res. Commun.* 182: 974, 1992.

New, M. I., White, P. C., Pang, S., Dupont, B., and Speiser, P. W. The adrenal hyperplasias. C. R. Scriver, A. L. Beaudet, W. S. Sly, and D. Valle (Eds.). *The Metabolic Basis of Inherited Disease.* New York: McGraw-Hill, 1989, Vol. II, Chap. 74, p. 1881.

Pascoe, L., Curnow, K. M., Slutsker, L., Rösler, A., and White, P. C. Mutations in the human *CYP11B2* (aldosterone synthase) gene causing corticosterone methyloxidase II deficiency. *Proc. Natl. Acad. Sci. USA* 89, 4996, 1992.

Picco, P., Garibaldi, L., Cotellessa, M., DiRocco, M., and Borrone, C. Corticosterone methyl oxidase type II deficiency: a cause of failure to thrive and recurrent dehydration in early infancy. *Eur. J. Pediatr.* 151: 170, 1992.

Rösler, A., and White, P. C. Mutations in human 11β-hydroxylase genes: 11β-hydroxylase deficiency in Jews of Morocco and corticosterone methyloxidase II deficiency in Jews of Iran. *J. Steroid Biochem. Mol. Biol.* 45: 99, 1993.

Answer 46

a. The symptoms suggest that there may be low levels of testosterone, as is indeed the case. If circulating levels of dehydroepiandrosterone, testosterone, and Δ^4-androstenedione are low, it is likely that one of the enzymes involved in their biosynthesis from other steroids is low. Three enzymes are closely involved in the biosynthesis of these compounds; a deficiency in any of these could result in lower testosterone levels. The enzyme 17β-hydroxysteroid dehydrogenase converts Δ^4-androstenedione into testosterone. Clearly, this could not be defective or there would be normal or greater levels of Δ^4-androstenedione. The enzyme 3β-hydroxysteroid dehydrogenase converts dehydroepiandrosterone into Δ^4-androstenedione. Again, if this were defective, then levels of dehydroepiandrosterone should be high. The enzyme *17,20 lyase* converts 17-hydroxypregnenolone into dehydroepiandrosterone and 17-hydroxyprogesterone into Δ^4-androstenedione. Since testosterone is made from Δ^4-androstenedione, a defect in 17,20 lyase would inhibit its synthesis as well as that of dehydroepiandrosterone and Δ^4-androstenedione. Hence the defective enzyme must be *17,20 lyase*.

Defects in earlier enzymes in the pathway, such as 17-hydroxylase, would also inhibit testosterone biosynthesis but would lower the levels of 17-hydroxypregnenolone and 17-hydroxyprogesterone as well as

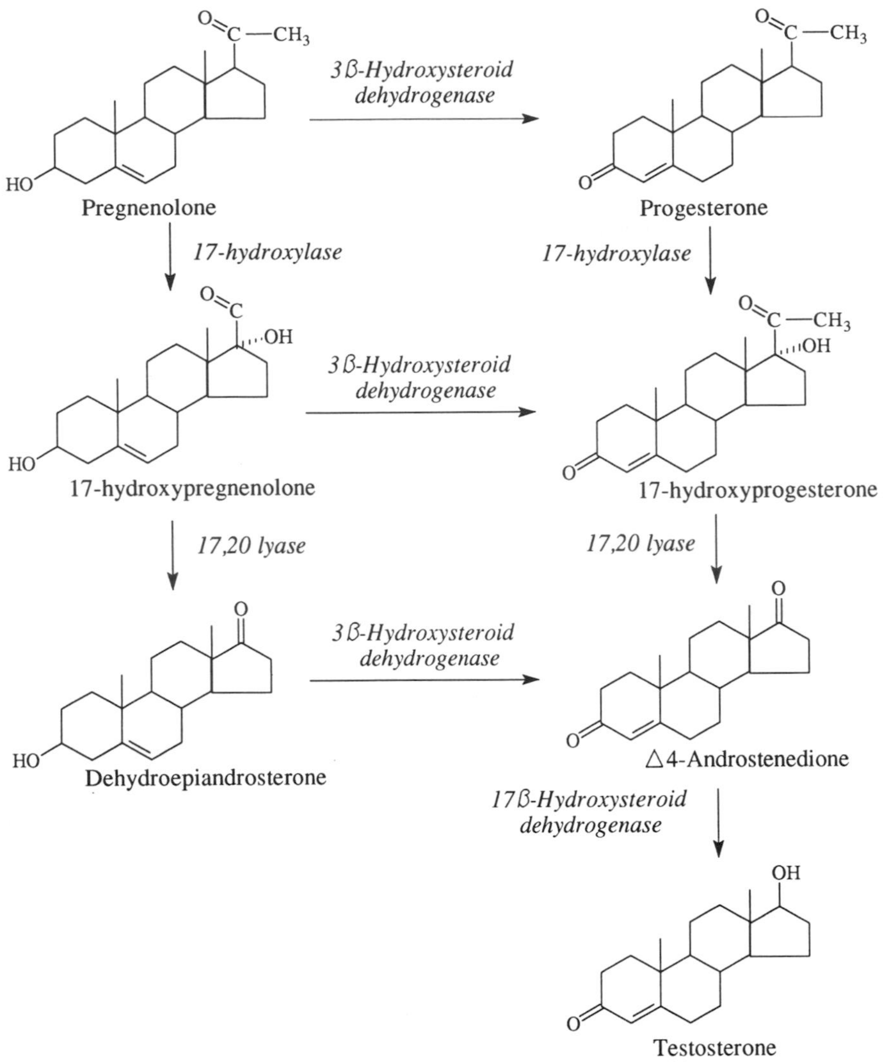

FIGURE A46-1. **Conversion of pregnenolone to testosterone.**

of the other three steroids. We are not told that these steroids are abnormally low.

b. See Figure A46-1.

c. The enzyme is cytochrome P450c17, which contains heme, which reacts with cyanide.

Your patient has ADRENAL HYPERPLASIA.

References

New, M. I., White, P. C., Pang, S., Dupont, B., and Speiser, P. W. The adrenal hyperplasias. C. R. Scriver, A. L. Beaudet, W. S. Sly, and D. Valle (Eds.). *The Metabolic Basis of Inherited Disease*. New York: McGraw-Hill, 1989, Vol. II, Chap. 74, p. 1881.

Smith, E. L., Hill, R. L., Lehman, I. R., Lefkowitz, R. J., Handler, P., and White, A. *Principles of Biochemistry: Mammalian Biochemistry*. New York: McGraw-Hill, 1983, p. 502.

Answer 47

a. Your patient has low circulating levels of all steroids, except for cholesterol. This implies that the defect is in some enzyme between cholesterol and the other steroids. Since your patient clearly has trouble converting cholesterol into pregnenolone, the defective enzyme is likely to be *cholesterol 20,22 desmolase*, which catalyzes the three steps of this reaction (Figure A47-1). The three activities of this enzyme are called 20α-hydroxylase, 22R-hydroxylase, and 20αR-dihydroxycholesteroliso-capronaldehyde-lyase. Since conversion of 20α-hydroxycholesterol into pregnenolone is normal, the defect must be in the part of the enzyme system that catalyzes the 20α-hydroxylase reaction. The low circulating levels of sodium imply low aldosterone production, since aldosterone works to raise sodium concentration. This is yet another of the steroids made in lowered amounts in this disease.

b. The enzyme is a cytochrome P450scc, which contains heme and therefore is inhibited by cyanide.

c. See Figure A47-1.

Your patient has LIPOID ADRENAL HYPERPLASIA.

References

Degenhart, H. J., Visser, H. K. A., and Boon, H. A study of the cholesterol splitting enzyme system in normal adrenals and in adrenal lipoid hyperplasia. *Acta Paediatr. Scand.* 60: 611, 1971.

ANSWER 47

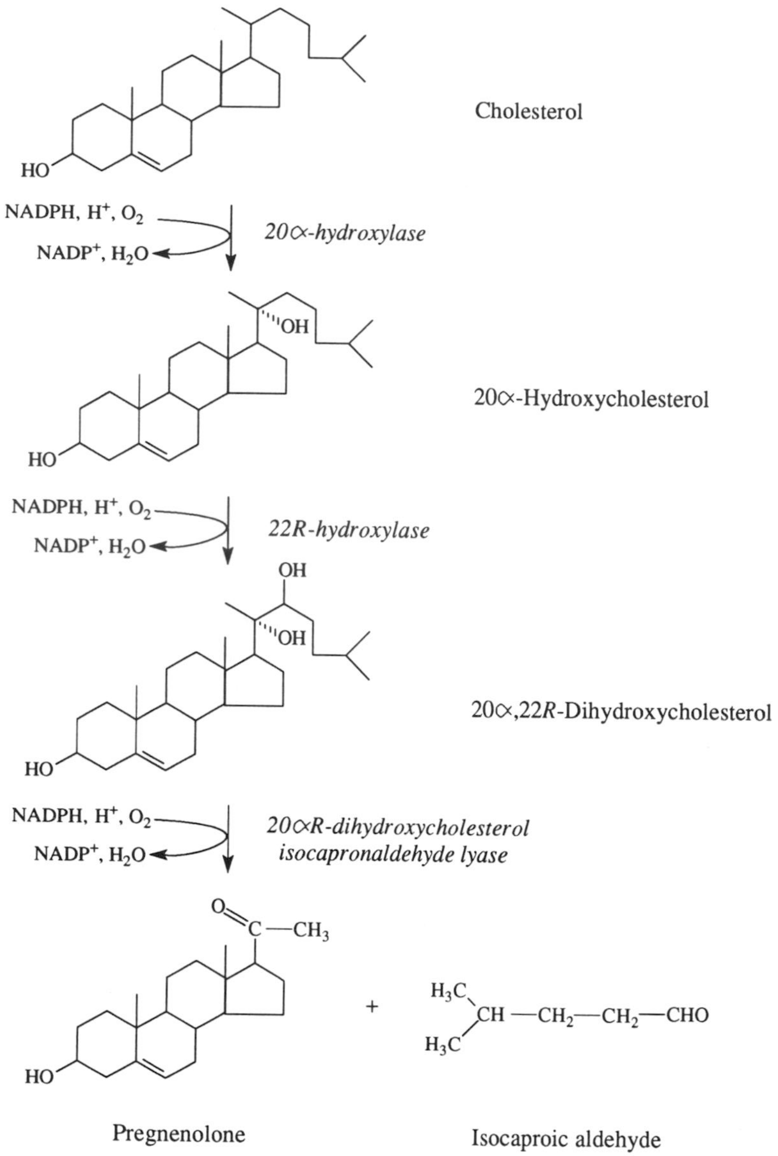

Cholesterol
HO
NADPH, H+, O2
NADP+, H2O
20α-hydroxylase
OH
20α-Hydroxycholesterol
HO
NADPH, H+, O2
NADP+, H2O
22R-hydroxylase
OH
OH
20α,22R-Dihydroxycholesterol
HO
NADPH, H+, O2
NADP+, H2O
20αR-dihydroxycholesterol
isocapronaldehyde lyase
O
C —CH3
+
H3C
CH —CH2—CH2—CHO
H3C
HO
Pregnenolone
Isocaproic aldehyde

FIGURE A47-1. **Cholesterol 20,22 desmolase reaction.**

Prader, A., and Gurtner, H. P. Das Syndrom des Pseudohermaphroditismus masculinus bei kongenitaler nebennierenrinden-Hyperplasie ohne Androgenüberproduktion (adrenaler Pseudohermaphroditismus masculinus). *Helv. Paediatr. Acta* 10: 397, 1955.

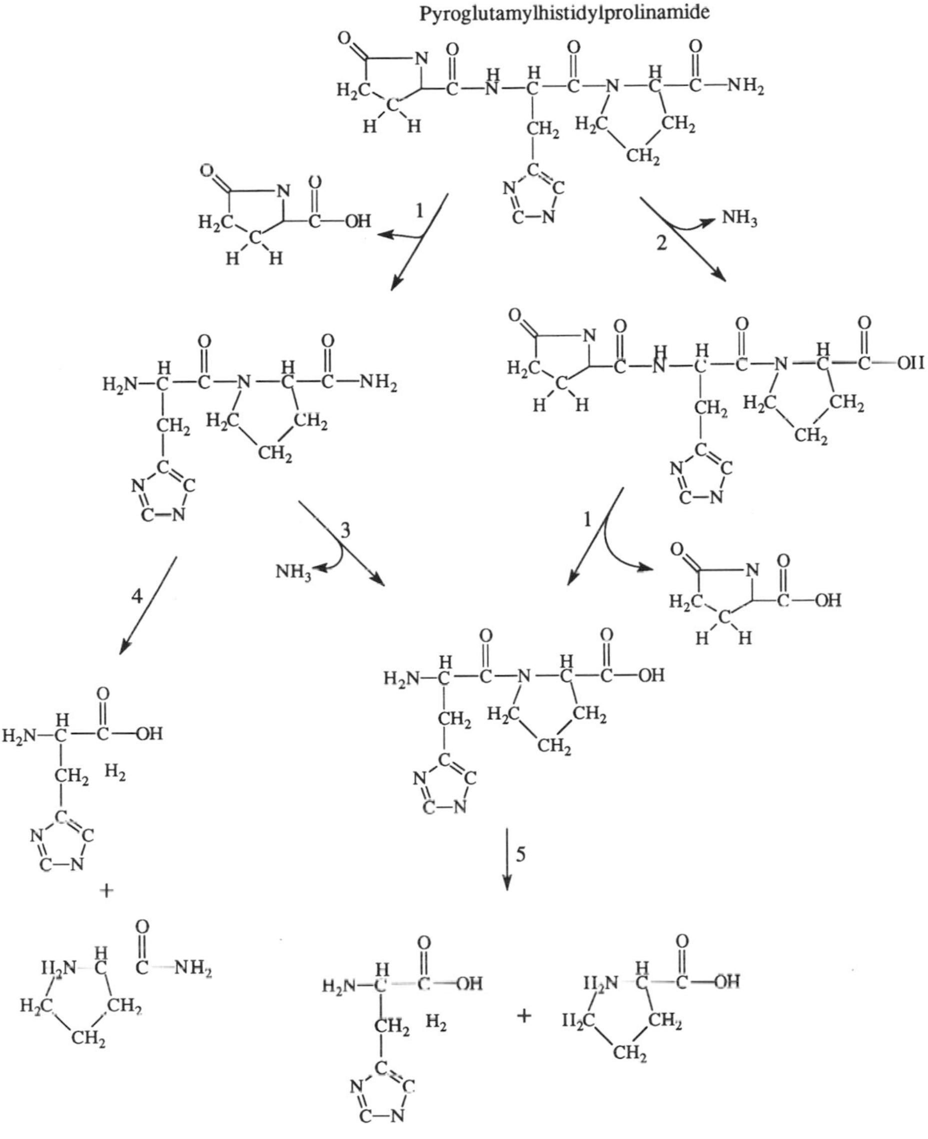

FIGURE A48-1. **Catabolism of TRH in the brain. Enzymes are as follows:
1, pyroglutamyl aminopeptidase, type I; 2, post proline cleaving endopeptidase;
3, dipeptidyl endopeptidase; 4, imidopeptidase; 5, proline dipeptidase.**

Answer 48

a. Pyroglutamylhistidylprolinamide, a tripeptide, is also known as thyrotropin-releasing hormone (TRH) (Figure 44-1).

b. Thyrotropin-releasing hormone (TRH) stimulates the pituitary to secrete thyroid-stimulating hormone. This hormone in turn stimulates the thyroid to secrete thyroxine and triiodothyronine. If the thyrotropin-releasing hormone is not cleared quickly from the blood, it is either not being degraded or, less likely, it does not encounter its receptor. The latter possibility can be eliminated because if it were true, we would see very little thyroid-stimulating hormone. Hence the defect must be in the degradation of thyrotropin-releasing hormone. The metabolism of TRH is complex. In the blood, TRH is degraded by the enzyme *pyrogluta-myl aminopeptidase, type II*. What happens to the resulting fragments in the blood is not clear. There is some evidence which suggests that triiodothyronine enhances activity of this enzyme in the blood, which would make sense as a kind of negative feedback control. In the brain, metabolism of TRH is more complex (Figure A48-1).

References

Fuse, Y., Polk, D. H., Lam, R. W., Reviczky, A. L., and Fisher, D. A. Distribution and ontogeny of thyrotropin-releasing hormone degrading enzymes in rats. *Am. J. Physiol.* 259: E787, 1990.

O'Cuinn, G., O'Connor, B., and Elmore, M. Degradation of thyrotropin-releasing hormone and luteinising hormone-releasing hormone by enzymes of brain tissue. *J. Neurochem.* 54: 1, 1990.

Suen, C.-S., and Wilk, S. Regulation of thyrotropin releasing hormone degrading enzymes in rat brain and pituitary by L-3,5,3'-triiodothyronine. *J. Neurochem.* 52: 884, 1989.

Yamada, M., and Mori, M. Thyrotropin-releasing hormone-degrading enzyme in human serum is classified as type II of pyroglutamyl aminopeptidase: influence of thyroid status. *Proc. Soc. Exp. Biol. Med.* 194: 346, 1990.

Answer 49

a. The defective enzyme must be the one that converts testosterone to dihydrotestosterone. This is *5α-reductase*, which catalyzes the reaction shown in Figure A49-1. Two forms of 5α-reductase exist in humans; only 5α-reductase 2 has so far been discovered to have mutations.

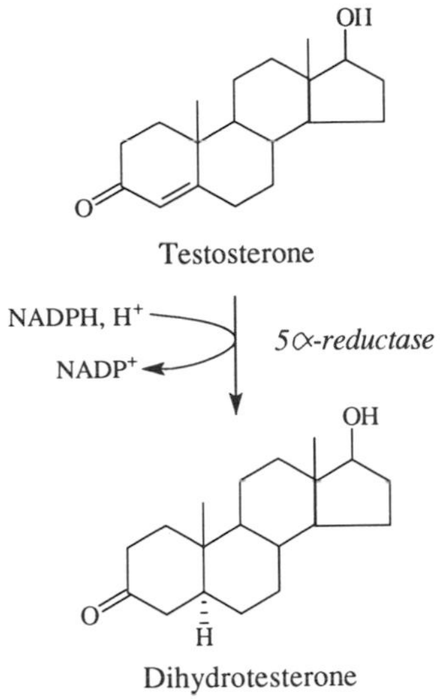

FIGURE A49-1. **5α-Reductase reaction.**

b. Male sex hormones work as follows. When testosterone enters a target cell, some of it is transformed by 5α-reductase into dihydrotestosterone. Both testosterone and dihydrotestosterone complex with the receptor protein. Both of these complexes bind to regions of the DNA and activate them. The two complexes have different effects, perhaps denoting different DNA binding sites. The testosterone-receptor complex induces formation of the epididymis and inner genitalia. The dihydrotestosterone-receptor complex is involved in formation of the external genitalia. External virilization is due to the action of the receptor complexed with dihydrotestosterone.

c. The defective enzyme, 5α-reductase 2, is normally expressed in many tissues that respond to testosterone. The other enzyme, 5α-reductase 1, so far has been found to be expressed in the prostate; it may be expressed in other tissues as well. During embryonic development, when testosterone is targeting certain tissues, if the 5α-reductase present in those tissues is only type 2 and if it is defective, dihydrotestosterone will not be produced in those tissues and development of those tissues will be defective. This cannot be compensated by having an equivalent, although functional enzyme present in another tissue.

d. Your patient's 5α-reductase 2 has an arginine at position 34 instead of a glycine. This could cause major differences in the structure of the enzyme. Glycine has essentially no side chain. It is often located where two segments of the polypeptide backbone are close together. Glycine could be located either on the surface or in the interior of a protein. By contrast, arginine is bulky and highly charged and is generally located on the exterior of a protein unless it is engaged in an ionic bond. We cannot tell exactly what changes the mutation has caused in the structure of your patient's enzyme, but it is clear that the V_{max} value of your patient's enzyme is considerably lower, as is its affinity for testosterone. Since the testosterone levels in cells are generally low, a decreased affinity for testosterone is a serious problem.

References

Andersson, S., and Russel, D. W. Structural and biochemical properties of clones and expressed human and rat steroid 5α-reductases. *Proc. Natl. Acad. Sci. USA* 87: 3640, 1990.

Griffin, J. E., and Wilson, J. D. The androgen resistance syndromes: 5α-reductase deficiency, testicular feminization, and related disorders. C. R. Scriver, A. L. Beaudet, W. S. Sly, D. Valle (Eds.). *The Metabolic Basis of Inherited Disease.* New York: McGraw-Hill, 1989, Vol. II, Chap. 75, p. 1919.

Thigpen, A. E., Davis, D. L., Gautier, T., Imperato-McGinley, J., and Russell, D. W. Brief report: the molecular basis of steroid 5α-reductase deficiency in a large Dominican kindred. *New Engl. J. Med.* 327: 1216, 1992.

Thigpen, A. E., Davis, D. L., Milatovich, A., Mendonca, B. B., Imperato-McGinlay, J., Griffin, J. E., Francke, U., Wilson, J. D., and Russell, D. W. Molecular genetics of steroid 5α-reductase 2 deficiency. *J. Clin. Invest.* 90: 799, 1992.

Answer 50

a. The male genitalia develop through the action of testosterone and of dihydrotestosterone in target cells. Dihydrotestosterone is formed by the action of 5α-reductase. Both testosterone and dihydrotestosterone bind to the same receptor, which then interacts with the DNA to activate certain genes. The specific genes that are activated depend on which androgen is bound to the receptor. During embryonic development, testosterone stimulates the development of the internal male genitalia, while dihydrotestosterone stimulates that of the external genitalia. Your patient has a disruption somewhere in this pathway. Since he is able to convert testosterone to dihydrotestosterone, the enzyme 5α-reductase, which catalyzes this conversion, must be normal. The inability of the radioactive dihydrotestosterone to localize to the nucleus suggests that there is an abnormality with the receptor. In the absence of a receptor, the dihydrotestosterone might drift randomly around the cell and not affect gene expression.

b. The complex of dihydrotestosterone and receptor binds to specific places on the nuclear DNA and activates certain genes which are responsible for virilization. If the receptor is defective, these genes will never be expressed.

c. First, identify the mutation:

Codon number: 713 714 715 716 717 718 719 720 721 722
Your patient:
   DNA: CAC GTG GTC AAG TGA GCC AAG GCC TTG CCT
   RNA: CAC GUG GUC AAG UGA GCC AAG GCC UUG CCU
   Protein: His Val Val Lys STOP
Normal person:
   DNA: CAC GTG GTC AAG TGG GCC AAG GCC TTG CCT
   RNA: CAC GUG GUC AAG UGG GCC AAG GCC UUG CCU
   Protein: His Val Val Lys Trp Ala Lys Ala Leu Pro

Your patient's androgen receptor has a nonsense mutation introduced into position 717 of the amino acid sequence. These are generally very serious mutations. The androgen receptor has three domains. The N-terminal domain, of unknown function, has a very unusual sequence, containing, among other oddities, a run of 20 consecutive glutamines, one of 8 prolines, and one of 23 glycines. The second domain binds to DNA. The third domain binds to either testosterone or dihydrotestosterone. The premature termination codon is in the third domain. Hence the ability of the receptor to bind to androgen is abolished. That is the primary defect, although without bound androgen, the receptor is unlikely to bind to DNA as well.

Your patient has COMPLETE ANDROGEN INSENSITIVITY.

References

Griffin, J. E. Androgen resistance: the clinical and molecular spectrum. *New Engl. J. Med.* 326: 611, 1992.

Griffin, J. E., and Wilson, J. D. The androgen resistance syndromes: 5α-reductase deficiency, testicular feminization, and related disorders. C. R. Scriver, A. L. Beaudet, W. S. Sly, and D. Valle (Eds.). *The Metabolic Basis of Inherited Disease.* New York: McGraw-Hill, 1989, Vol. II, Chap. 75, p. 1919.

Lubahn, D. B., Brown, T. R., Simental, J. A., Higgs, H. N., Migeon, C. J., Wilson, E. M., and French, F. S. Sequence of the intron/exon junctions of the coding region of the human androgen receptor gene and identification of a point mutation in a family with complete androgen insensitivity. *Proc. Natl. Acad. Sci. USA* 86: 9534, 1989.

Sai, T., Seino, S. Chang, C., Trifiro, M., Pinsky, L., Mhatre, A., Kaufman, M., Lambert, B., Trapman, J., Brinkmann, A. O., Rosenfield, R. L., and Liao, S. An exonic point mutation of the androgen receptor gene in a family with complete androgen insensitivity. *Am. J. Hum. Genet.* 46: 1095, 1990.

Answer 51

a. African pygmies do not respond to injections of human growth hormone with an increase in insulin-like growth factor I. This would suggest that either pygmies have fewer receptors for growth hormone or that they are unable to make insulin-like growth factor I. However, the fact that pygmies have normal levels of insulin-like growth factor I prior to puberty suggests that this is not the case. The likely situation is that pygmies do not have enhanced production of growth hormone receptor at puberty, indicating that a likely role of the steroid sex hormones, which cause many changes during puberty, is to enhance the production of growth hormone receptor.

b. Insulin-like growth factor I is also called somatomedin C; it is a 70-amino acid peptide. Its amino acid sequence is related to that of proinsulin. It has various biological activities, including stimulating the growth of cartilage, synthesis of collagen and glycosaminoglycans, uptake of glucose, and cell division.

References

Phillips, J. A. Inherited defects in growth hormone synthesis and action. C. R. Scriver, A. L. Beaudet, W. S. Sly, and D. Valle (Eds.). *The Metabolic Basis of Inherited Disease.* New York: McGraw-Hill, 1989, Vol. II, Chap. 77, p. 1965.

Phillips, L. S., and Vassilopoulou-Sellin, R. Somatomedins. *New Engl. J. Med.* 302: 371, 1980.

Answer 52

a. Your patient has elevated parathyroid hormone in his blood, yet appears to have the symptoms of an underactive parathyroid (low calcium, high phosphate). The logical deduction is that your patient has a problem with the signal transduction mechanism for parathyroid hormone. The experiment with the kidney biopsy confirms this deduction; since addition of parathyroid hormone does not result in increased cAMP production, there is clearly a problem in signal transduction. In principle, this problem could be in the receptor protein itself, in the G protein components, or in the adenyl cyclase. The observation that cAMP production is normal in response to both thyroid-stimulating hormone and glucagon suggests that it is specific for parathyroid hormone and therefore must involve the *parathyroid hormone receptor* itself.

b. Here we are considering a different set of circumstances. What if your patient's biopsy samples had made little cAMP in response to either parathyroid hormone, thyroid-stimulating hormone, or glucagon? This would imply a more general defect. In this case the defect would not be in a specific receptor but in some part of the signal transduction system that mediates or regulates the outcome of the hormonal signal. One likely candidate would be *adenyl cyclase,* the enzyme that converts ATP to cAMP. Since cholera toxin is able to ADP-ribosylate the G_s protein, the results of your experiment suggest that the G_s protein is normal in your patient. However, it is also possible that the G_i protein is abnormal in your patient, is overly active, and hence is able to overinhibit production of cAMP.

Your patient has PSEUDOHYPOPARATHYROIDISM TYPE Ib.

Reference

Spiegel, A. M. Pseudohypoparathyroidism. C. R. Scriver, A. L. Beaudet, W. S. Sly, and D. Valle (Eds.). *The Metabolic Basis of Inherited Disease.* New York: McGraw Hill, 1989, Vol. II, Chap. 79, p. 2013.

Answer 53

a. The traditional cause of rickets is lack of vitamin D, which in a normal person is produced by the action of ultraviolet light. It can also be a dietary supplement. Vitamin D is metabolized to its fully active form 1α,25-dihydroxycholecalciferol by the scheme shown in Figure A53-

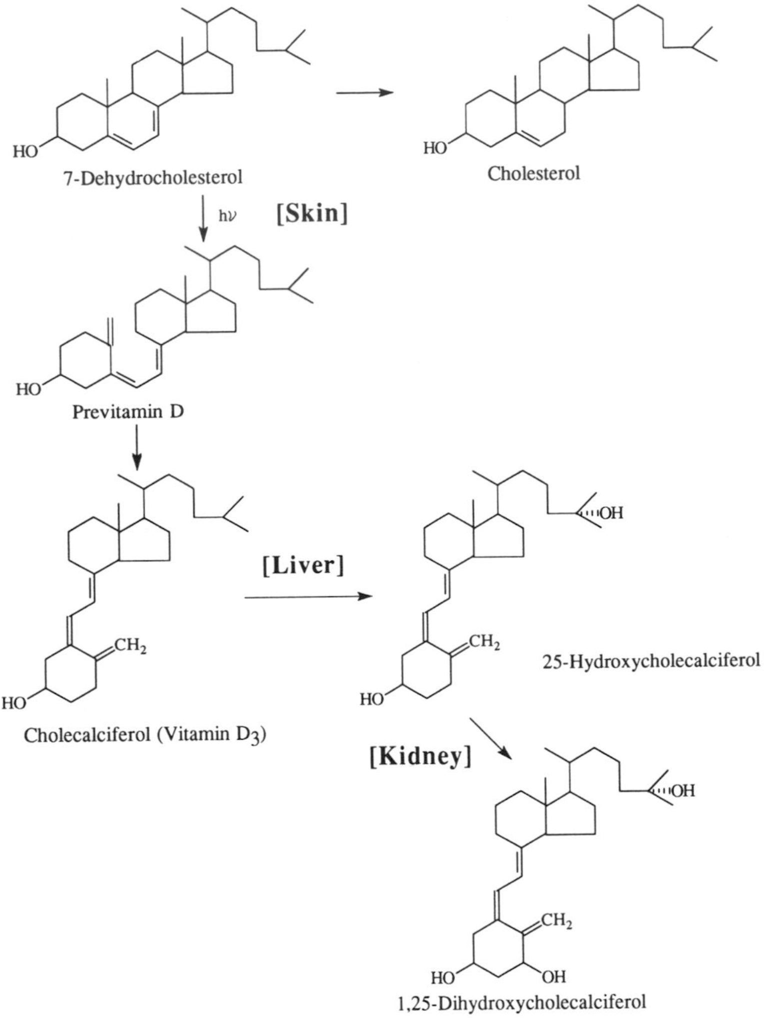

FIGURE A53-1. **Biosynthesis of 1α,25-dihydroxycholecalciferol.**

1. The calcium-mobilizing effects of vitamin D are mediated by $1\alpha,25$-dihydroxycholecalciferol. Your patient clearly has normal levels of $1\alpha,25$-dihydroxycholecalciferol in his blood, but the calcium levels are low, implying that the $1\alpha,25$-dihydroxycholecalciferol is unable to act, or, in other words, that there is a problem with the *$1\alpha,25$-dihydroxycholecalciferol receptor*. The fact that elevated doses of $1\alpha,25$-dihydroxycholecalciferol can alleviate the problem is consistent with this hypothesis.

b. Since higher concentrations of $1\alpha,25$-dihydroxycholecalciferol can saturate the receptors on target cells to the same extent as would be true for a normal person, we must conclude that there is no problem in the number of receptors but rather that their affinity for $1\alpha,25$-dihydroxycholecalciferol is lower than normal.

Reference

Marx, S. J. Vitamin D and other calciferols. C. R. Scriver, A. L. Beaudet, W. S. Sly, and D. Valle (Eds.). *The Metabolic Basis of Inherited Disease*. New York: McGraw-Hill, 1989, Vol. II, Chap. 80, p. 2029.

Answer 54

a. From the nucleotide sequence one can predict the amino acid sequence as follows:

Codon number:	59	60	61
Your patient:			
DNA:	ACA	GCT	GAG
RNA:	ACA	GCU	GAG
Protein:	Thr	Ala	Glu
Normal person:			
DNA:	ACA	ACT	GAG
RNA:	ACA	ACU	GAG
Protein:	Thr	Thr	Glu

Thus your patient's transthyretin has an alanine at position 60, where a normal person has a threonine. Alanine is considerably more hydrophobic than threonine. Since position 60 is on the outside of the protein, it is likely that the introduction of a hydrophobic amino acid at this position could lead to aggregation, especially since this protein exists as a tetramer; the tetrameric nature of transthyretin means that this mutation would introduce four hydrophobic spots onto the surface of the protein. Aggregation is certainly likely. This is analogous to sickle cell anemia, in which the replacement of a glutamate with a valine residue in the β subunit introduces a hydrophobic residue onto the surface and leads to aggregation.

b. Transthyretin, formerly called prealbumin, is a plasma protein that transports thyroxine and retinol. Transthyretin exists as a tetramer. The subunits of the tetramer are arranged such that there is a channel in the middle in which thyroxine binds. Retinol does not bind directly to thyretin. First, retinol binds to retinol-binding protein, which then binds to the outside of the transthyretin tetramer. The retinol-binding protein will not bind to transthyretin in the absence of retinol.

Your patient has PREALBUMIN AMYLOIDOSIS.

Reference

Benson, M. D., and Wallace, M. R. Amyloidosis. C. R. Scriver, A. L. Beaudet, W. S. Sly, and D. Valle (Eds.). *The Metabolic Basis of Inherited Disease.* New York: McGraw-Hill, 1989, Vol. II, Chap. 97, p. 2439.

Answer 55

a. The thyroid produces thyroxine and triiodothyronine in response to the hormone thyrotropin (thyroid-stimulating hormone, TSH). In the design of the experiment, thyrotropin is the most likely hormone to generate an effect. The defective protein must be in the pathway from thyrotropin to cAMP; in other words, the alteration must be in either the receptor, G protein, or adenyl cyclase. The defect is manifest in the absence of hormone. When hormone is present, both the active and inactive cells generate the same amount of cAMP (Table P55-2). In the absence of hormone, the inactive cells generate less cAMP than do the active cells. The sequence of the altered protein is quite revealing. If you convert Table P55-1 as Table A55-1, you will see a large region

TABLE A55-1

Region	Length of Segment	Percent Hydrophobic Residues	Location with Respect to Membrane
1	415	48	Outside
2	25	88	Transmembrane
3	10	30	Inside
4	23	78	Transmembrane
5	21	48	Outside
6	22	59	Transmembrane
7	21	52	Inside
8	23	87	Transmembrane
9	21	57	Outside
10	24	79	Transmembrane
11	20	35	Inside
12	23	78	Transmembrane
13	13	54	Outside
14	20	80	Transmembrane
15	83	42	Inside

with relatively few hydrophobic residues, followed by regions that are alternately high and low in hydrophobic residues. The regions with high hydrophobicity are 20 to 25 residues long and are likely to be transmembrane segments. The N-terminal region has five potential glycosylation sites (Asn-X-Ser and Asn-X-Thr) and hence is likely to be an extracellular domain. A protein that has an extracellular domain and transmembrane segments is not likely to be either a G protein or an adenyl cyclase. Hence the altered protein is *thyrotropin receptor.*

b. The active gene must be the mutant and the inactive gene is the normal form. Here is the reason. Imagine if the inactive cells were the mutant. Then the active cells should be generating normal amounts of thyroid hormone. Nevertheless, your patient is hyperthyroid. Hence the active gene must be mutated. Also, there is no difference in the response of the active and inactive cells to thyrotropin. The difference is their cAMP production in the absence of hormone. cAMP production leads to thyroid hormone secretion. If the inactive cells were the mutants, the normal cells would always be producing thyroid hormone even in the absence of thyrotropin, and this does not make good regulatory sense. Hence the mutation must be one that keeps the thyrotropin receptor partially "turned on" even in the absence of thyrotropin.

To figure out the nature of the mutation, we can analyze it as follows:

Residue number:	619	620	621	622	623	624	625	626	627	628	629	630
Active cells:												
DNA:	GAC	ACC	AAG	ATT	ATC	AAG	AGG	ATG	GCC	GTG	TTG	ATC
mRNA:	GAC	ACC	AAG	AUU	AUC	AAG	AGG	AUG	GCC	GUG	UUG	AUC
Protein:	Asp	Thr	Lys	Ilu	Ilu	Lys	Arg	Met	Ala	Val	Leu	Ilu
Inactive cells:												
DNA:	GAC	ACC	AAG	ATT	GCC	AAG	AGG	ATG	GCC	GTG	TTG	ATC
mRNA:	GAC	ACC	AAG	AUU	GCC	AAG	AGG	AUG	GCC	GUG	UUG	AUC
Protein:	Asp	Thr	Lys	Ilu	Ala	Lys	Arg	Met	Ala	Val	Leu	Ilu

This is a rare type of mutation in which two adjacent nucleotide residues (GC) have mutated to AU. The result is that alanine is replaced by isoleucine at position 623. In which region of the protein is position 623? Table P55-1 tells us that it is in region 11. Assuming that region 1 is extracellular (a reasonable assumption in view of the glycosylation sites), region 11 must be intracellular. The intracellular portions of the receptor are the ones where the receptor interacts with G protein. The alanine in the normal protein occurs in this small region that has relatively few hydrophobic residues. In the mutant, the alanine is replaced with a significantly larger hydrophobic residue, isoleucine. Presumably, in the normal protein, the binding of thyrotropin to the receptor causes a conformational change that affects region 11 so as to alter its interaction with G protein. Conceivably, the orientation of the polypeptide backbone is altered as part of this change. The alanine at position 623 may not have any particular role to play, but replacing it by a bulkier residue may automatically alter the position of the polypeptide backbone to one more closely resembling the one that ensues upon binding of thyrotropin to the receptor. The result would be a system that is always at least partially active; its activity is to stimulate the thyroid cells to proliferate and to produce the thyroid hormones. Hence your patient will have elevated concentrations of thyroid hormone and the symptoms of hyperthyroidism.

Why do we see both genes in the same person? The reason is that this is not an inherited, but rather a somatic mutation. Since one of the functions of the thyrotropin receptor is to mediate proliferation, a somatic mutation that results in activating the gene all the time will result in proliferation and formation of clones with the altered gene. Thus the mutant thyrotropin receptor is acting like an oncogene. Cells that have normal genes will not proliferate. Thus both genes will be expressed.

c. The cells that make the normal gene are essentially inactive and not making thyroid hormone. The reason is that the excess activity of the mutant cells causes increased concentrations of thyroid hormones in the blood. Both triiodothyronine and thyroxine inhibit secretion of thyrotropin by the pituitary; in addition, triiodothyronine inhibits secretion of thyrotropin-releasing hormone from the hypothalamus (thyrotropin-releasing hormone stimulates the pituitary to produce thyrotropin). The result is that thyroid hormone inhibits production of thyrotropin. Your patient will thus have very low circulating concentrations of thyrotropin. Thus the normal cells will not be stimulated to produce thyroid hormone and will be inactive. The mutant cells, in contrast, do not need thyrotropin to be active.

Your patient has HYPERFUNCTIONING THYROID ADENOMA.

References

Akamizu, T., Ikuyama, S., Saji, M., Kosugi, S., Kozak, C., McBride, O. W., and Kohn, L. D. Cloning, chromosomal assignment, and regulation of the rat thyrotropin receptor: expression of the gene is regulated by thyrotropin, agents that increase cAMP levels, and thyroid autoantibodies. *Proc. Natl. Acad. Sci. USA* 87: 5677, 1990.

Kosugi, S., Okajima, F., Ban, T., Hidaka, A., Shenker, A., and Kohn, L. D. Mutation of alanine 623 in the third cytoplasmic loop of the rat thyrotropin (TSH) receptor results in a loss in the phosphoinositide but not cAMP signal induced by TSH and receptor autoantibodies. *J. Biol. Chem.* 267: 24153, 1992.

Parma, J., Duprez, L., Van Sande, J., Cochaux, P., Gervy, C., Mockel, J., Dumont, J., and Vassart, G. Somatic mutations in the thyrotropin receptor gene cause hyperfunctioning thyroid adenomas. *Nature* 365: 649, 1993.

Answer 56

a. The enzyme you tested must be the one that converts 18-hydroxycorticosterone into aldosterone. The enzyme is *18-hydroxy dehydrogenase*, also known as aldosterone synthase or corticosterone methyl oxidase II.

b. The 5' regulatory region of 11β-hydroxylase attached to the gene for 18-hydroxydehydrogenase means that the 18-hydroxy dehydrogenase will be made wherever the 11β-hydroxylase is normally expressed, such as in the zona fasciculata. Also, since the regulatory factor for 11β-hydroxylase is ACTH, the ACTH will enhance production of 18-hydroxy dehydrogenase by these cells.

c. Glucocorticoids, as part of a normal feedback mechanism, inhibit synthesis of ACTH. By lowering ACTH levels, they also decrease production of the chimeric aldosterone gene product; hence there will be less aldosterone produced.

Your patient has GLUCOCORTICOID-REMEDIATED ALDOSTE-RONISM.

References

Chu, M. D., and Ulick, S. Isolation and identification of 18-hydroxycortisol from the urine of patients with primary aldosteronism. *J. Biol. Chem.* 257: 2218, 1982.

Gomez-Sanchez, C. E., Montgomery, M., Ganguly, A., Holland, O. B., Gomez-Sanchez, E. P., Grim, C. E., and Weinberger, M. H. Elevated urinary excretion of 18-oxocortisol in glucocorticoid-suppressible aldosteronism. *J. Clin. Endocrinol. Metab.* 59: 1022, 1984.

Lifton, R. P., Dluhy, R. G., Powers, M., Rich, G. M., Cook, S., Ulick, S., and Lalouel, J.-M. A chimaeric 11β-hydroxylase/aldosterone synthase gene causes glucocorticoid-remediable aldosteronism and human hypertension. *Nature* 355: 262, 1992.

New, M. I., and Peterson, R. E. A new form of congenital adrenal hyperplasia. *J. Clin. Endocrinol. Metab.* 27: 300, 1967.

Simpson, E. R., and Waterman, M. R. Regulation of the synthesis of steroidogenic enzymes in adrenal cortical cells by ACTH. *Annu. Rev. Physiol.* 50: 427, 1988.

Sutherland, D. J. A., Ruse, J. L., and Laidlaw, J. C. Hypertension, increased aldosterone secretion and low plasma renin activity relieved by dexamethasone. *Can. Med. Assoc. J.* 95: 1109, 1966.

Ulick, S., Chan, C. K., Gill, J. R., Gutkin, M., Letcher, L., Mantero, F., and New, M. I. Defective fasciculata zone function as the mechanism of glucocorticoid-remediable aldosteronism. *J. Clin. Endocrinol. Metab.* 71: 1151, 1990.

Ulick, S., Chu, M. D., and Land, M. Biosynthesis of 18-oxocortisol by aldosterone-producing adrenal tissue. *J. Biol. Chem.* 258: 5498, 1983.

CHAPTER 9

The Blood

Problem 57

Your patient is a 30-year-old man with a tendency to develop thromboembolism. Your tests reveal that he has a deficiency of active protein S.

a. How does this deficiency explain the tendency to develop thromboembolism?

b. You do a liver biopsy and do the following assay. You add $^{14}CO_2$ and vitamin K and measure the incorporation of ^{14}C into protein S and prothrombin. You find that incorporation into protein S is 50% of normal while that into prothrombin is normal. Suppose also that the molecular weight of your patient's protein S is normal (70 kD). What would this result tell you about the nature of the defect in your patient's protein S?

c. Write out the reaction in which vitamin K participates and the cycle that regenerates the vitamin K.

Problem 58

Your patient has a tendency to bleed too much. He bruises easily, bleeds from his gums, and has severe bleeding when he has a tooth extracted. His circulating level of factor VIII is low. His level of factor V is normal. You observe that injecting him with factor VIII provides only limited protection from bleeding since the factor VIII in his blood seems unstable. You collect some of his blood, purify his platelets and his plasma, and do the following test. You add the antibiotic ristocetin, which induces platelet aggregation, and measure the extent of aggregation. The results are listed in Table P58-1.

You find that a certain protein is altered at position 550. Where a normal person's DNA has a TGG codon at this position, your patient has a TGC codon. You purify the altered protein and measure its ability to interact with platelet glycoprotein Ib. You do the experiment by measuring the ability of the protein to compete for binding with an antibody to glycoprotein Ib. You add 2 μM concentrations of protein and measure how much radioactive antibody remains bound to platelet preparation. You obtain the results listed in Table P58-2.

a. What is the protein likely to be defective in your patient? What is the role of this protein?

b. Describe the biosynthesis of this protein.

c. What is the mutation in your patient? What might it do to the structure of the protein? From the results of the binding experiment, explain how the symptoms of the disease arise in your patient.

TABLE P58-1

Source of Platelets	Source of Plasma	Aggregation (% of control)
Normal person	Normal person	100
Normal person	Your patient	20
Your patient	Normal person	100
Your patient	Your patient	20

TABLE P58-2

Source of Protein	Ristocetin Present	Amount of Antibody Bound (%)
No protein	n/a	100
Normal person	No	100
Normal person	Yes	35
Your patient	No	5
Your patient	Yes	0

Problem 59

Your patient has a tendency to bleed too much. He bruises easily, bleeds from his gums, and has severe and prolonged bleeding when he has a tooth extracted. You observe that his blood contains giant platelets, about the size of his erythrocytes. His circulating levels of factor V and VIII are normal. You collect some of his blood, purify his platelets and his plasma, and do the following test. You add the antibiotic ristocetin, which induces platelet aggregation, and measure the extent of aggregation. The results are listed in Table P59-1.

You use antibodies to purify two of his membrane glycoproteins, glycoprotein Ib and glycoprotein IX. You subject these proteins to polyacrylamide gel electrophoresis in the presence of sodium dodecyl sulfate and find that glycoprotein Ib from your patient migrates the same as glycoprotein Ib from a normal person. However, glycoprotein IX from your patient migrates as several species. In addition to a band at the normal molecular weight of about 140 kD, there are two additional bands of 115 kD and 105 kD; these bands are not seen in the glycoprotein IX of a normal person.

You are able to clone the gene for the α chain of glycoprotein Ib from your patient. You see one difference in the sequence:

Codon number:	54	55	56	57	58	59	60
Your patient:	TAC	ACT	CGC	TTC	ACT	CAG	CTG
Normal person:	TAC	ACT	CGC	CTC	ACT	CAG	CTG

a. What are the roles of glycoprotein Ib and glycoprotein IX?

b. How might the mutation explain the results, including the results obtained on the gels?

TABLE P59-1

Source of Platelets	Source of Plasma	Aggregation (% of control)
Normal person	Normal person	100
Normal person	Your patient	100
Your patient	Normal person	20
Your patient	Your patient	20

Problem 60

Two of your patients, George and Edward, are botany professors specializing in the history of the human use of plants. While traveling together in Italy, they recalled that in the sixth century B.C., the philosopher Pythagoras had warned his followers against eating fava beans (*Vicia faba*). George recalled that he had eaten fava beans before without any problem, so he was convinced that Pythagoras was wrong. He persuaded Edward to join him in consuming some cooked fava beans. Although Edward ate fewer beans than George, he became quite ill. He became very pale, severely anemic, and somewhat jaundiced. He also exhibited a massive hemoglobinuria. He would have died had he not received a blood transfusion in Naples. When you saw Edward again, you told him that you could have predicted his reaction to fava beans based on his very similar reaction to the antimalarial prophylactic you had prescribed for him 10 years before when he was about to embark on an expedition to the Amazon.

a. Which of Edward's enzymes is defective?

b. How does the normal functioning of this enzyme protect the erythrocytes?

Problem 61

Your patient is a 22-year-old man who appears cyanotic. He reports frequent headaches and a tendency to become easily fatigued and out of breath when he exercises. You draw his blood, which is brownish in color. It does not become red even when you shake it with air. You purify his erythrocytes as well as some fibroblasts and do a radioimmunoassay with an antibody specific for cytochrome b_5 reductase. You find that your patient has very low levels of cytochrome b_5 reductase in his erythrocytes, although the level in other tissues appears to be normal.

When you sequence the gene of your patient's cytochrome b_5 reductase, you find the following:

Codon number:	55	56	57	58	59
Your patient:	GAC	ACC	CAG	CGC	TTC
Normal person:	GAC	ACC	CGC	CGC	TTC

You do an experiment in which you examine the protein's ability to survive either heat treatment or trypsin digestion. The results are listed in Table P61-1.

How do these findings account for the symptoms? Describe the electron transfer pathway in which this protein is involved.

TABLE P61-1

	Activity Remaining (%)	
Source of Protein	Heating at 50°C, 80 min	Trypsin, 30 min
Normal person	80	00
Your patient	40	20

Problem 62

Your patient is a 13-month-old girl who appears cyanotic. She also exhibits severe mental retardation and microcephaly. After her death, autopsy reveals incomplete myelinization of her nerves and a cerebroside content in her brain about 50% of the normal. She also had decreased content of unsaturated fatty acids and increased palmitate in her adipose tissue. Just before she died, you gave her some methylene blue, which improved her color but did nothing for her other symptoms. You do a radioimmunoassay with an antibody specific for cytochrome b_5 reductase and find that the level of cytochrome b_5 reductase in your patient's erythrocytes and other tissues is low.

a. How does this defect account for the low level of unsaturated fatty acids?

b. How did the methylene blue make your patient less cyanotic?

Problem 63

Your patient has an enlarged and painful spleen; she exhibits recurrent vomiting, jaundice, and episodes of losing her voice. Her muscles are weak. Many of her erythrocytes are spherical in shape. Such erythrocytes are destroyed in the spleen. You purify some of your patient's erythrocytes and lyse them. From the resulting erythrocyte "ghosts" you extract the proteins. When you examine the spectrin by polyacrylamide gel electrophoresis, you find that the α and β bands are present in lower concentrations and so is the ankyrin band. You obtain a sample of your patient's reticulocytes and measure mRNA contents. You find that the mRNAs for α- and β-spectrin are present in normal amounts, but ankyrin mRNA is present at 50% of normal amounts. How do these findings account for the unusual shape of the erythrocytes?

Problem 64

Your patient has an enlarged spleen and has frequent headaches. She appears to be chronically weak. Many of her erythrocytes are ellipsoidal or even rod-shaped. There is excess lysis of the erythrocytes. When you analyze spectrin from her erythrocytes by polyacrylamide gel electrophoresis, you find that the β chain is significantly smaller. The α chain is normal. You are able to sequence the gene for β-spectrin from your patient and from a normal person and you find the sequences in the end of the gene coding for the C-terminal region of β-spectrin. The β-spectrin gene for a normal person has the following structure (nucleotides in exons are capitalized; those in introns are lowercase; codon divisions are entered in the exons):

```
        Exon W                                    Exon X (197 nu)
GAG CGG CTC CGC ATG Tgtgag . . . ggcagTG CTG GAG GTG . . . CCC ACC ACG gtgag . . .

        Exon Y (50 nu)                            Exon Z (145 nu)
tctag CTT GAC CTG . . . GAG ACT GGgtgag . . . cttagG CCT CAA GAG GAG . . . TAC TAG
```

When you compare the sequence of your patient's β-spectrin gene with that of a normal person, you find the following:

Your patient: CCCACCACGgtgggg

Normal person: CCCACCACGgtgag

You construct a cDNA from the mRNA for your patient's β-spectrin. The partial sequence is as follows:

GAGCGGCTCCGCATGTCTTGAGCTG . . . .

Note: "nu" stands for nucleotides; ". . ." means a sequence that is not specified.

a. How many amino acids shorter is your patient's β-spectrin than that of normal β-spectrin? What is the C-terminal residue of your patient's β-spectrin?

b. How could the observed defect lead to the abnormal erythrocytes?

Problem 65

The Chediak–Higashi syndrome is a disease in which the patients have numerous severe infections and usually die in their first decade. If you scrape their skin and put a microscope slide on the scraped area (the "skin window" test), very few leukocytes appear, indicating that their motility is poor. The leukocytes of these patients are full of giant granules. Although tubulin is normal in these leukocytes, there appears to be a deficiency in microtubule assembly. Imagine that you find that you can get leukocyte tubulin from a Chediak–Higashi patient to assemble normally in vitro by adding brain microtubule-associated proteins.

a. What would you conclude is the deficiency in the Chediak–Higashi patient?

b. How would a deficiency in microtubule assembly account for the poor motility and giant granules?

Problem 66

Your patient has recurrent infections, particularly fungal and bacterial. Many of the infections involve the skin and the respiratory or gastrointestinal systems. You find that your patient's leukocytes respond to chemotactic factors by increasing their motility, just as do those of normal patients. You purify the leukocytes and you do an experiment in which you compare the response of your patient's leukocytes and those of a normal person after addition of a chemotactic peptide. You find that in your patient's leukocytes, normal amounts of inositol-1,4,5-trisphosphate are produced and intracellular proteins are phosphorylated to a normal extent. However, you find that no $NADP^+$ is produced, nor is H_2O_2 produced. You find that one of your patient's genes, which codes for a 91-kD protein, has a different sequence, as follows:

Codon number:	414	415	416
Your patient:	ACA	CAC	TTC
Normal person:	ACA	CCC	TTC

a. Name the defective enzyme and describe its structure. What is the reaction that it catalyzes?

b. How does this defect prevent killing of bacteria?

Problem 67

Your patient is normally healthy except for a susceptibility to *Candida* infections. His leukocytes appear to be normal in their morphology. You purify the leukocytes and you do an experiment in which you compare the response of your patient's leukocytes and those of a normal person after addition of a chemotactic peptide. You find that the production of $NADP^+$ and H_2O_2 is a little higher than normal. However, very little hypochlorite (HOCl) is produced.

a. Name the defective enzyme and describe the reaction that it catalyzes.

b. How does this defect prevent killing of organisms such as fungi?

Problem 68

Your patient is a 5-year-old girl with recurrent infections. She has frequent infections on her skin, infections that never develop pus but which crater and leave scars after treatment. She has had appendicitis and often has milder gastrointestinal infections. She has frequent earaches and sinusitis as well as severe gum disease. If you scrape her skin and put a microscope slide on her scraped area (the "skin window" test), virtually no leukocytes appear on the slide. You find that her leukocytes are motile but unable to adhere to endothelial cells as would leukocytes from a normal patient. You draw some blood and separate the leukocytes. You find that when you add dead bacteria bound to C3b, the leukocytes do not phagocytize them. You purify the leukocyte membranes and solubilize them and analyze them by polyacrylamide gel electrophoresis. You find that your patient's leukocytes are lacking a glycoprotein called β or CD18.

a. How does this lack account for the symptoms?

b. You have another patient, with similar but milder symptoms, whose leukocytes lack the membrane glycoprotein αL (also known as CD11a). Assuming that this was their only deficiency, would you expect these leukocytes to adhere to dead bacteria bound to C3b? Why or why not?

Answer 57

a. Protein S in an accelerating factor in the reaction by which activated protein C cleaves and inactivates factors Va and VIIIa. The latter two are large proteins that play critical roles in accelerating the proteolytic activations of prothrombin and factor X, respectively. By destroying factors Va and VIIIa, activated protein C can regulate the rate of blood coagulation. If protein S is defective, it will be unable to stimulate the protein C reaction, and hence the concentrations of factors Va and VIIIa will rise and this will in turn increase the tendency to clot and form emboli. Deficiencies in protein S are likely to be serious; they can predispose to cerebral infarction.

b. A carboxyl group is added to the γ carbon of certain glutamate residues in protein S as well as other blood coagulation factors (factors VII, IX, X, prothrombin, and protein C) in a vitamin K–dependent reaction that occurs in the liver; such a modified residue is called γ-carboxyglutamate. The extra carboxyl groups permit the factor to chelate with calcium and orient properly with respect to the platelet membrane. If the labeled $^{14}CO_2$ is not being incorporated into your patient's protein S in the presence of vitamin K, there is a problem with the formation of γ-carboxyglutamate residues in protein S. In principle, the problem could be with the carboxylation system in the liver, consisting of vitamin K epoxidase, vitamin K epoxide reductase, and vitamin K dehydrogenase. However, if that were the case, prothrombin would not incorporate ^{14}C label either and we are informed that it does. Hence the problem must be with protein S. It is unlikely that there has been a deletion of the region which contains the glutamate residues which become carboxylated because the apparent molecular weight has not changed significantly. Normal protein S contains 11 residues of γ-carboxyglutamate. It is hard to imagine a mutation other than a deletion, or a frameshift, which would affect five or six glutamate residues simultaneously. Thus one possibility is a frameshift mutation which alters a region with five or six glutamate residues. Another possibility is a change in the conformation of the protein which makes the glutamate residues less accessible to the carboxylating system.

c. The carboxylation reaction is shown in Figure A57-1 and vitamin K regeneration in Figure A57-2.

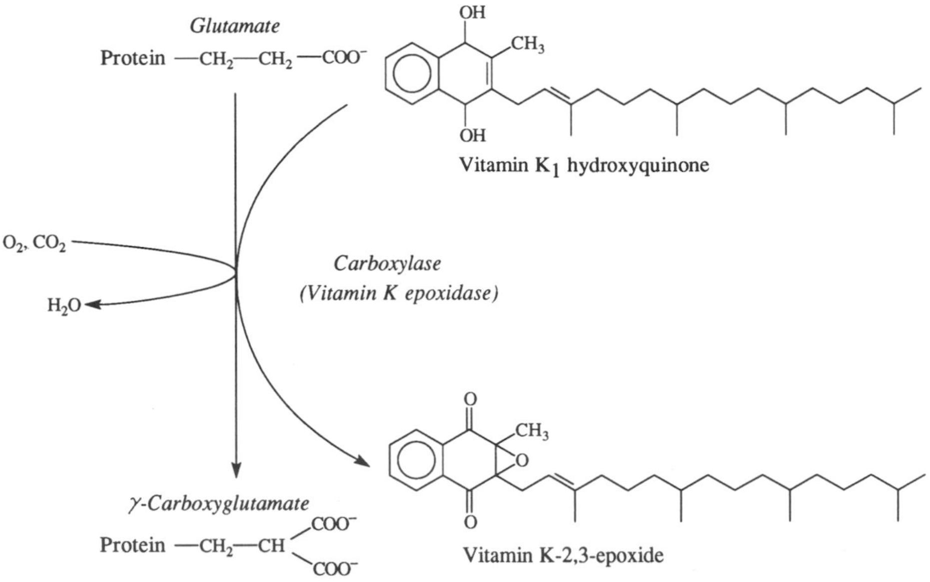

FIGURE A57-1. **Vitamin K–dependent γ-carboxylation of protein-bound glutamate. In this figure, vitamin K$_1$ is shown; this is the form of vitamin K made by green plants. Only one of its isoprenoid units has a double bond. Bacteria (such as those in the gut) produce vitamin K$_2$, in which each isoprenoid unit (which can vary from 1 to 15) contains a double bond.**

References

Devilat, M., Toso, M., and Morales, M. Childhood stroke associated with protein C or S deficiency and primary antiphospholipid syndrome. *Pediatr. Neurol.* 9: 67, 1993.

Rich, C., Gill, J. C., Wernick, S., and Konkol, R. J. An unusual cause of cerebral venous thrombosis in a four-year-old child. *Stroke* 24: 603, 1993.

Silverman, R. B., and Nandi, D. L. Reduced thioredoxin: a possible physiological cofactor for vitamin K epoxide reductase. Further support for an active site disulfide. *Biochem. Biophys. Res. Commun.* 155: 1248, 1988.

Uotila, L. The metabolic functions and mechanism of vitamin K. *Scand. J. Clin. Lab. Invest.* 50, Suppl. 201: 109, 1990.

Whitlon, D. S., Sadowski, J. A., and Suttie, J. W. Mechanism of coumarin action: significance of vitamin K epoxide reductase inhibition. *Biochemistry* 17: 1371, 1978.

Answer 58

a. Your patient has a form of hemophilia. This can be caused by a defect in the production or activity of any of several blood coagulation

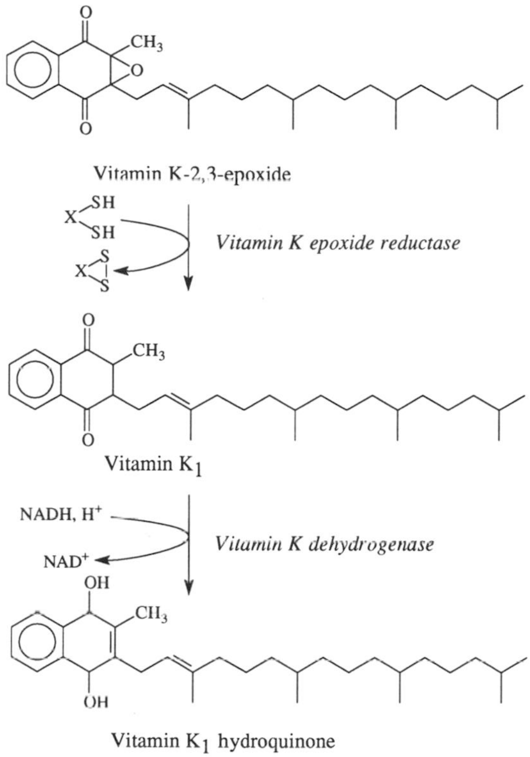

FIGURE A57-2. **Regeneration of vitamin K hydroquinone. The vitamin K epoxide reductase requires a dithiol to carry out the reaction. The bearer of the dithiol (X in the figure) has not been identified, but lipoic acid and thioredoxin are good candidates. Vitamin K epoxide reductase is very sensitive to the anticoagulant warfarin. The vitamin K dehydrogenase reaction can be carried out by two different enzymes, one of which is sensitive to warfarin and one that is insensitive.**

factors. Deficiency in factor VIII is one of the most common and is associated with the famous classical or royal hemophilia. Your patient has low circulating levels of factor VIII, which would at first cause you to suspect a defect in the synthesis or structure of your patient's factor VIII. However, you find that your patient seems to degrade injected factor VIII very rapidly compared to a normal person. This would not be the case if he simply had a defect in factor VIII. The experiment in which you measured platelet aggregation using both platelets and plasma from a normal person as well as your patient indicated that the defect is likely to be in some soluble factor that would bind to platelets to induce them to aggregate. The factor would also stabilize factor VIII. There is a factor that does these things: the *von Willebrand factor.*

Von Willebrand factor has two major roles. One is to bind to and stabilize factor VIII to prevent it from being prematurely degraded. A second role is to mediate platelet adhesion to subendothelial surfaces, such as collagen. These surfaces would become exposed when a blood vessel is damaged. By helping bind the platelets to these surfaces, von Willebrand factor helps to localize the platelets and the platelet-mediated coagulation factors to the damaged area. A series of binding sites have been identified on the von Willebrand factor. There are two sites that bind to factor VIII (with affinities of 5 to 7 $\times$ 10^{-11} M and 3 to 5 $\times$ 10^{-10} M). There is one site that binds to glycoprotein Ib (a platelet surface protein) if the platelet is activated by thrombin or ristocetin (Figure A58-1). There is a site for binding collagen and one for binding to platelet glycoproteins IIb and IIIa. These binding sites allow von Willebrand factor to anchor platelets to collagen surfaces and to speed up the coagulation process by stabilizing factor VIII.

b. Von Willebrand factor has a very complex biosynthesis. It is synthesized in endothelial cells and megakaryocytes. As the megakaryocytes mature into platelets, the mature von Willebrand factor is stored in the platelets. The steps in biosynthesis are as follows:

1. Von Willebrand factor is synthesized on the ribosomes as a polypeptide of 2813 amino acids.

2. In the process of transfer to the endoplasmic reticulum, the 22-amino acid signal peptide is removed by a signal peptidase.

3. In the endoplasmic reticulum, the von Willebrand factor is glycosylated at 12 asparagines and 10 serines and threonine. The von Willebrand factors dimerize by disulfide bond formation between their C-terminal regions.

4. In the Golgi, the oligosaccharides are processed. The N-linked oligosaccharides are complex type. The O-linked oligosaccharides are tetrasaccharides consisting of two sialic acids, one galactose and one N-acetylgalactosamine.

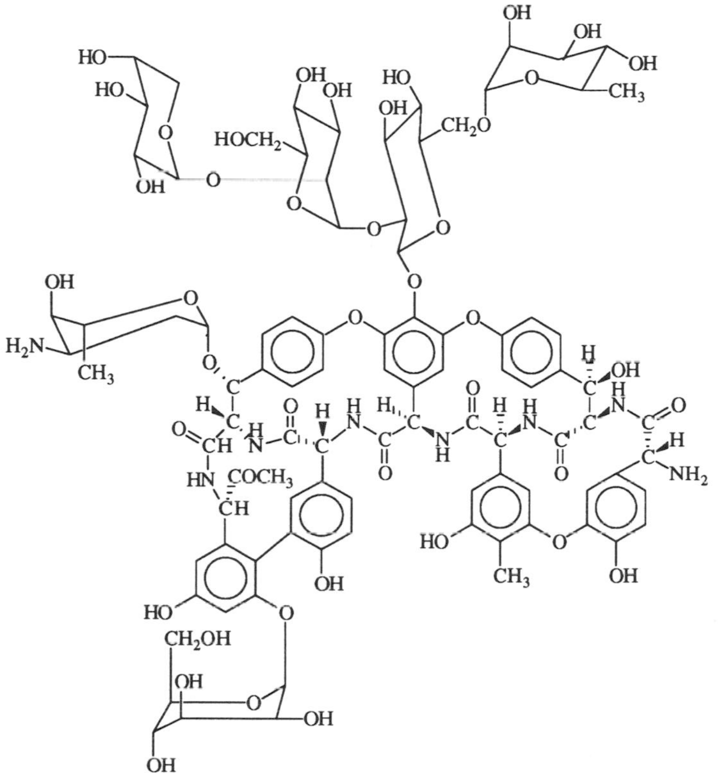

FIGURE A58-1. **Structure of ristocetin.**

5. Some of the oligosaccharides are sulfated.

6. The von Willebrand factor dimers now form multimers by formation of disulfide bridges. There can be up to 20 monomers in the multimer, forming a structure that can be 1.3 μm long. The multimeric form is more active than the dimeric form.

7. In the secretory granule, a peptide of 741 amino acids is removed from the N-terminal. The function of this peptide is unknown. These secretory granules are also known as Weibel–Palade bodies.

8. Von Willebrand factor is secreted in two ways. The majority is secreted constitutively as a mixture of different size multimers. The second pathway, stimulated by agents such as thrombin, acts on the Weibel–Palade bodies; the secreted von Willebrand factor is now in the form of the largest multimer. This is the most potent form of von Willebrand factor.

9. In the serum, there is a protease that cleaves von Willebrand between Tyr^{842} and Met^{843} and diminishes its activity.

   c. The mutation in the von Willebrand protein is readily identified. The codon TGG becomes UGG upon transcription and codes for tryptophan. The codon TGC becomes UGC and codes for cysteine. Thus your patient has a cysteine at position 550 in his von Willebrand factor instead of a tryptophan. This position is in the domain that binds glycoprotein Ib; therefore, it is not surprising that it would affect binding to this protein. Tryptophan is a hydrophobic amino acid that would tend to be buried in a protein; cysteine has a tendency to form disulfides. In a protein such as this, which is rich in cysteines and disulfides, the introduction of a new cysteine may disrupt the disulfide bridge pattern, leading to major changes in the overall structure.
   The results of the binding experiment are illuminating. When the normal protein is added to platelets in the absence of ristocetin, the antibody is not displaced; this means that normal von Willebrand factor will not bind to glycoprotein Ib in the absence of ristocetin. However, in the presence of ristocetin, about 65% of the antibody is displaced. Ristocetin mimics the effect of thrombin. It activates the platelets to permit glycoprotein Ib to bind to von Willebrand factor. The results you obtain with the normal von Willebrand factor are precisely what you would expect. In your patient's protein, however, you see a different pattern. In the absence of ristocetin, your patient's von Willebrand factor displaces 95% of the antibody, and in the presence of ristocetin, it displaces 100% of the antibody. In other words, your patient's von Willebrand factor binds much better to glycoprotein Ib than does the normal von Willebrand factor. At first, it may seem counterintuitive that this should cause a problem. However, the most significant result of your binding experiment is that your patient's von Willebrand factor should bind to platelets at all in the absence of ristocetin. Normally, von Willebrand factor is not supposed to bind to platelets except when the platelets are activated by thrombin, which is released during coagulation. That your patient's von Willebrand factor should bind to platelets at any time is very ominous. It means that your platelets will be clearing von

Willebrand factor out of the circulation and that when you need it, it will not be there. This would lead to the bleeding disorder.

Your patient has TYPE IIB VON WILLEBRAND DISEASE.

References

Budavari, S. *The Merck Index: An Encyclopedia of Chemicals, Drugs, and Biologicals*, 11th Ed. Rahway, NJ: Merck & Co., Inc., 1989, p. 1311.

Coney, K. A., Nichols, W. C., Bruck, M. E., Bahou, W. F., Shapiro, A. D., Bowie, E. J. W., Gralnick, H. R., and Ginsburg, D. The molecular defect in type IIB von Willebrand disease. *J. Clin. Invest.* 87: 1227, 1991.

Ganz, P. R., Atkins, J. S., Palmer, D. S., Dudani, A. K., Hashemi, S., and Luison, F. Definition of the affinity of binding between human von Willebrand factor and coagulation factor VIII. *Biochem. Biophys. Res. Commun.* 180: 231, 1991.

Lynch, D. C. The fine structure of von Willebrand factor multimers and von Willebrand disease. *Ann. N.Y. Acad. Sci.* 614: 138, 1991.

Mayadas, T. N., and Wagner, D. D. Von Willebrand factor biosynthesis and processing. *Ann. N.Y. Acad. Sci.* 614: 153, 1991.

Ruggeri, Z. M., and Ware, J. The structure and function of von Willebrand factor. *Thromb. Haemostasis* 67: 594, 1992.

Sadler, J. E. Von Willebrand disease. C. R. Scriver, A. L. Beaudet, W. S. Sly, and D. Valle (Eds.). *The Metabolic Basis of Inherited Disease.* New York: McGraw-Hill, 1989, Vol. II, Chap. 87, p. 2171.

Sadler, J. E., Mancuso, D. J., Randi, A. M., Tuley, E. A., and Westfield, L. A. Molecular biology of von Willebrand factor. *Ann. N.Y. Acad. Sci.* 614: 114, 1991.

Samor, B., Michalski, J. C., Mazurier, C., Goudemand, M., De Waard, P., Vliegenthart, J. F., Strecker, G., and Montreuil, J. Primary structure of the major O-glycosidically linked carbohydrate unit of human von Willebrand factor. *Glycoconjugate J.* 6: 263, 1989.

Ware, J., Dent, J. A., Azuma, H., Sugimoto, M., Kyrle, P. A., Yoshioka, A., and Ruggeri, Z. M. Identification of a point mutation in type IIB von Willebrand disease illustrating the regulation of von Willebrand factor affinity for the platelet membrane glycoprotein Ib–IX receptor. *Proc. Natl. Acad. Sci. USA* 88: 2946, 1991.

Weiss, H. J. Von Willebrand factor and platelet function. *Ann N.Y. Acad. Sci.* 614: 125, 1991.

Answer 59

a. Your test tells you that the defect is in the platelets and not in the plasma. Hence the defective factor or factors is not a soluble one, but one inside the platelet or part of the platelet membrane. Glycoprotein Ib and glycoprotein IX are such platelet proteins. Glycoprotein Ib is the receptor for von Willebrand factor. Von Willebrand factor is a protein that stabilizes factor VIII and mediates adhesion between platelets and subendothelial surfaces. For von Willebrand factor to carry out the latter role, it must bind to the platelets, and its receptor on the platelet membrane is glycoprotein Ib. A defect in glycoprotein Ib could lead to poor platelet binding to subendothelial surfaces and hence to increased bleeding.

b. You need to identify the mutation:

Codon number:	54	55	56	57	58	59	60
Your patient:							
DNA:	TAC	ACT	CGC	TTC	ACT	CAG	CTG
RNA:	UAC	ACU	CGG	UUC	ACU	CAG	CUG
Protein:	Tyr	Thr	Arg	Phe	Thr	Gln	Leu
Normal person:							
DNA:	TAC	ACT	CGC	CTC	ACT	CAG	CTG
RNA:	UAC	ACU	CGC	CUC	ACU	CAG	CUG
Protein:	Tyr	Thr	Arg	Leu	Thr	Gln	Leu

Your patient has a phenylalanine at position 57 where a normal person would have a leucine. Superficially, this would seem to be a relatively innocuous mutation, since both phenylalanine and leucine are hydrophobic amino acids with a tendency to be on the interior of proteins. In this case the picture is more complicated. The amino acid sequence of glycoprotein Ibα has six leucine-rich imperfect repeats. The first of these in the sequence is residues 47 to 70. The leucine at position 57 is conserved in every one of these repeats, as is the leucine at position 60. Although the precise role of the leucine is not known, the fact that it is conserved in all of these repeats (including one repeat in the β subunit) suggests that substitutions are deleterious. Often, this type of sequence occurs in polypeptide chains that form α helices that are associated with other α helices. Even though we cannot be certain as to the exact role of Leu[57], it is likely that a mutation at this position would cause inappropriate arrangement of the polypeptide chains.

At this point we have to recall the results obtained with the gel electrophoresis. The protein that looked abnormal there was glycoprotein

IX; glycoprotein Ib migrated normally. It looked as if glycoprotein IX had been partly proteolyzed; that would account for the presence of bands of lower molecular weight. How could a mutation in glycoprotein Ib affect the susceptibility to proteolysis of glycoprotein IX? The answer is that your patient's mutation in glycoprotein Ib is likely to affect its association with other polypeptide chains. It is likely that those polypeptide chains are those of glycoprotein IX. Perhaps the mutation in glycoprotein Ib weakens its association with glycoprotein IX, thereby exposing the latter and making it more susceptible to proteolysis. Glycoprotein Ib and glycoprotein IX must therefore be associated. The proper arrangement of the ensemble is probably required for von Willebrand factor to bind to glycoprotein Ib. In your patient's case, the ensemble is defective and hence von Willebrand factor binds less well.

Your patient has BERNARD–SOULIER SYNDROME.

References

Lopez, J. A., Chung, D. W., Fujikawa, K., Hagen, F. S., Papayannopoulou, T., and Roth, G. J. Cloning of the α chain of human platelet glycoprotein Ib: a transmembrane protein with homology to leucine-rich α_2-glycoprotein. *Proc. Natl. Acad. Sci. USA* 84: 5615, 1987.

Miller, J. L., Lyle, V. A., and Cunningham, D. Mutation of leucine-57 to phenylalanine in a platelet glycoprotein Ibα leucine tandem repeat occurring in patients with an autosomal dominant variant of Bernard–Soulier disease. *Blood* 79: 439, 1992.

Roth, G. J. Developing relationships: arterial platelet adhesion, glycoprotein Ib, and leucine-rich glycoproteins. *Blood* 77: 5, 1991.

Answer 60

a. People who are sensitive to antimalarial drugs have a defect in the enzyme glucose-6-phosphate dehydrogenase. These people are also likely to be susceptible to divicine (2,4-diamino-5,6-dihydroxypyrimidine) and isouramil (4-amino-2,5,6-trihydroxypyrimidine), two pyrimidine derivatives found in fava beans. These compounds rapidly oxidize the erythrocytes' supply of glutathione. Reduced glutathione is involved in protecting membranes from oxidative damage. Reduced glutathione is a substrate for the enzyme glutathione peroxidase which converts H_2O_2 (hydrogen peroxide) to water; the enzyme glutathione reductase then

FIGURE A60-1. **Structures of divicine and isouramil.**

converts the oxidized glutathione produced by the glutathione peroxidase reaction back into reduced glutathione. If the reduced glutathione is oxidized by divicine and isouramil, glutathione peroxidase activity will decrease and the concentrations of H_2O_2 will remain high enough to damage the membranes. Divicine and isouramil (Figure A60-1) also appear to interact directly with sulfhydryl groups of membrane proteins, thereby altering the membrane structure and perhaps weakening it.

b. Glucose-6-phosphate dehydrogenase is a key enzyme in the pentose phosphate pathway. It transfers electrons from glucose-6-phosphate to NADPH. By generating NADPH, it keeps glutathione reduced, which protects erythrocytes against oxidative damage by H_2O_2, probably to membranes.

Edward has FAVISM. This is a disease common in Mediterranean countries, where fava beans are often eaten.

References

Arese, P., Bosia, A., Naitana, A., Gaetani, S., D'Aquino, M., and Gaetani, G. F. Effect of divicine and isouramil on red cell metabolism in normal and G6PD-deficient (Mediterranean variant) subjects: possible role in the genesis of favism. G. Brewer (Ed.). *The Red Cell: Fifth Ann Arbor Conference.* New York: Alan R. Liss, 1981, p. 725.

Budavari, S. *The Merck Index: An Encyclopedia of Chemicals, Drugs, and Biologicals,* 11th Ed. Rahway, NJ: Merck & Co., Inc., 1989, pp. 533–534.

Luzzatto, L., and Mehta, A. Glucose-6-phosphate dehydrogenase deficiency. C. R. Scriver, A. L. Beaudet, W. S. Sly, and D. Valle (Eds.). *The Metabolic Basis of Inherited Disease.* New York: McGraw-Hill, 1989, Vol. II, Chap. 91, p. 2237.

Answer 61

Cytochrome b_5 reductase is involved in the transfer of electrons from NADH or NADPH to hemoglobin (Figure A61-1). If hemoglobin inside the erythrocyte becomes oxidized so that the iron atom in the heme is in the $+3$ oxidation state, the heme no longer functions to transport

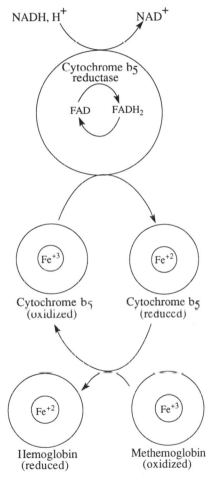

FIGURE A61 1. **Reduction of methemoglobin by cytochrome b_5 and cytochrome b_5 reductase.**

oxygen. Occasionally, for various reasons, some of our hemoglobin molecules become oxidized; to counter this eventuality, our erythrocytes contain this pathway aimed at reducing any oxidized hemoglobin back to the +2 (reduced) state, in which it can transport oxygen. In your patient's case, the deficiency is likely to be restricted to the enzyme in erythrocytes; this makes the disease less serious than it could be.

In your patient, the defect in cytochrome b_5 reductase leads to a hemoglobin that is partly nonfunctional; hence his tissues do not get the oxygen they need and he becomes easily fatigued and out of breath.

The mutation can be identified readily:

Codon number:	55	56	57	58	59
Your patient:					
DNA:	GAC	ACC	CAG	CGC	TTC
RNA:	GAC	ACC	CAG	CGC	UUC
Protein:	Asp	Thr	Gln	Arg	Phe
Normal person:					
DNA:	GAC	ACC	CGC	CGC	TTC
RNA;	GAC	ACC	CGC	CGC	UUC
Protein:	Asp	Thr	Arg	Arg	Phe

Your patient's protein has a glutamine instead of an arginine. Although both amino acids are polar, arginine is charged and can participate in ionic bonds, but glutamine cannot do so. We do not know if this arginine was involved in such bonds, but if it was, the mutant protein should be less stable than the normal protein. Indeed, the results of the experiment show that is indeed the case. The mutant protein is far less resistant to either trypsin or heat treatment than is the normal protein. This suggests that the problem with the protein is that the cytochrome b_5 reductase is unstable. This would shorten its lifetime and would produce a deficiency of the protein and of this electron transport pathway.

An interesting question is why the deficiency is restricted to the erythrocyte cytochrome b_5 reductase, since the same enzyme is associated with microsomes in many other tissues. The erythrocyte protein is smaller than the microsomal protein but is likely coded for by the same gene; probably the erythrocyte enzyme arises by processing. It is conceivable that there is a problem in the processing of the erythrocyte enzyme in your patient.

Your patient has ENZYMOPENIC HEREDITARY METHEMOGLO-BINEMIA, TYPE I.

References

Jaffé, E. R., and Hultquist, D. E. Cytochrome b_5 reductase deficiency and enzymopenic hereditary methemoglobinemia. C. R. Scriver, A. L. Beaudet, W. S. Sly, and D. Valle (Eds.). *The Metabolic Basis of Inherited Disease*. New York: McGraw-Hill, 1989, Vol. II, Chap. 92, p. 2267.

Shirabe, K., Yubisui, T., Borgese, N., Tang, C., Hultquist, D. E., and Takeshita, M. Enzymatic instability of NADH-cytochrome b_5 reductase as a cause of hereditary methemoglobinemia type I (red cell type). *J. Biol. Chem.* 267: 20416, 1992.

Answer 62

a. Cytochrome b_5 participates in the desaturation of fatty acids as part of the *NADH-dependent Δ^9-stearyl-CoA desaturase* system.

1. *Cytochrome b_5 reductase*

$$NADH + H^+ + FAD \rightarrow NAD^+ + FADH_2$$

$$FADH_2 + 2 \text{ cytochrome } b_5 \text{ (Fe}^{3+}) \rightarrow FAD + 2H^+ + 2 \text{ cytochrome } b_5 \text{ (Fe}^{2+})$$

2. *Desaturase*

$$2 \text{ cytochrome } b_5 \text{ (Fe}^{7+}) + R-CH_2-CH_2-(CH_2)_7-\overset{\overset{\displaystyle O}{\|}}{C}-CoA + O_2 + 2H^+ \rightarrow$$

$$2 \text{ cytochrome } b_5 \text{ (Fe}^{3+}) + R-CH=CH-(CH_2)_7-\overset{\overset{\displaystyle O}{\|}}{C}-CoA + 2H_2O$$

Hence lack of the enzyme may inhibit oxidation of fatty acids.

b. The cyanosis could be eased by methylene blue (Figure A62-1), which stimulates electron transport from NADPH to methemoglobin.

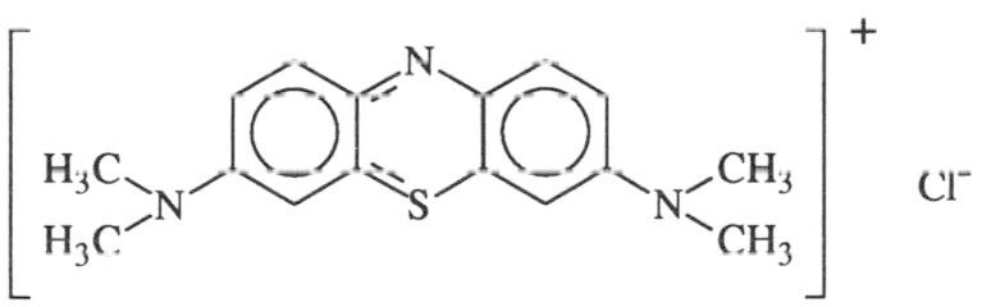

FIGURE A62-1. **Structure of methylene blue.**

This, however, would not affect the other consequences of the cytochrome b_5 reductase deficiency.

Your patient has ENZYMOPENIC HEREDITARY METHEMOGLO-BINEMIA, TYPE II.

References

Budavari, S. *The Merck Index: An Encyclopedia of Chemicals, Drugs, and Biologicals*, 11th Ed. Rahway, NJ: Merck & Co., Inc., 1989, p. 954.

Jaffé, E. R., and Hultquist, D. E. Cytochrome b_5 reductase deficiency and enzymopenic hereditary methemoglobinemia. C. R. Scriver, A. L. Beaudet, W. S. Sly, and D. Valle (Eds.). *The Metabolic Basis of Inherited Disease*. New York: McGraw-Hill, 1989, Vol. II, Chap. 92, p. 2267.

Leroux, A., Junien, C., Kaplan, J.-C., and Bamberger, J. Generalised deficiency of cytochrome b_5 reductase in congenital methaemoglobinaemia with mental retardation. *Nature* 258: 619, 1975.

Smith, E. L., Hill, R. L., Lehman, I. R., Lefkowitz, R. J., Handler, P., and White, A. *Principles of Biochemistry: General Aspects*. New York: McGraw-Hill, 1983, p. 374.

Answer 63

Spectrin is the major protein of the erythrocyte cytoskeleton, a network of proteins that underlies the erythrocyte membrane. Spectrin consists of two polypeptide chains: α (MW 240,000) and β (MW 220,000). Spectrin molecules polymerize to form fibers and also interact with other cytoskeletal proteins such as actin. They also bind to ankyrin. Ankyrin (202 to 206 kD) plays a key role in cytoskeletal architecture because, as its name might imply, it acts as an anchor, binding proteins such as spectrin or pallidin to integral membrane proteins. Since the mRNA levels of ankyrin are low while those of α- and β-spectrin are normal, we should conclude that the defect in ankyrin is primary. In other words, decreased ankyrin prevents much of the spectrin from binding to the erythrocyte membrane. In short, with a defect in ankyrin the numerous interactions that stabilize the erythrocyte cytoskeleton are disrupted. Therefore, the erythrocyte cannot retain its usual shape and can easily become spherical.

Your patient has HEREDITARY SPHEROCYTOSIS.

References

Bennett, V. Ankyrins. T. Kreis and R. Vale (Eds.). *Guidebook to the Cytoskeletal and Motor Proteins.* Oxford: Oxford University Press, 1993, p. 221.

Hanspal, M., Yoon, S.-H., Hanspal, J. S., Lambert, S., Palek, J., and Prchal, J. T. Molecular basis of spectrin and ankyrin deficiencies in severe hereditary spherocytosis: evidence implicating a primary defect of ankyrin. *Blood* 77: 165, 1991.

Lux, S. E., and Becker, P. S. Disorders of the red cell membrane skeleton: hereditary spherocytosis and hereditary elliptocytosis. C. R. Scriver, A. L. Beaudet, W. S. Sly, and D. Valle (Eds.). *The Metabolic Basis of Inherited Disease.* New York: McGraw-Hill, 1989, Vol. II, Chap. 95, p. 2367.

Peters, L. L., and Lux, S. E. Ankyrins: structure and function in normal cells and hereditary spherocytes. *Semin. Hematol.* 30: 85, 1993.

Answer 64

a. The mutation is in an intron. Such a mutation is likely to cause a splicing error:

> Your patient: CCCACCACGgtggg
> Normal person: CCCACCACGgtgag

To figure out how much shorter the β-spectrin is we have to identify the new splicing arrangement. By lining up the nucleotide sequence of the cDNA with the information given about the sequence of the β-spectrin gene in a normal person, it is possible to do this:

	Exon W	Exon X	Exon Y
Gene sequence:	GAG CGG CTC CGC ATG Tgt . . . agTG . . .	ACG gt . . .	ug CTT GAC CTG . . .
cDNA sequence:	GAG CGG CTC CGC ATG T		CTT GAG CTG . . .

You will notice that in the new splicing, all of exon X is deleted. You will also notice, however, that because the intron between exons W and X began in the middle of a codon, we have a frameshift in exons Y and Z. The amino acid sequence becomes the following:

cDNA: GAG CGG CTC CGC ATG TCT TGA GCT G . . .
RNA: GAG CGG CUC CGC AUG UCU UGA GCU G . . .
Protein: Glu   Arg   Leu   Arg   Met   Ser   STOP

You have therefore introduced a STOP codon near the beginning of exon Y. This means that none of exon Z is expressed and only one amino acid of exon Y. The new C-terminal amino acid is *serine.*

How much shorter is your patient's β-spectrin than that of a normal person?

All of exon X is removed:	197 nu
All of exon Y is removed, except for the first two nucleotides (the end of the serine codon) and the three nucleotides coding for the STOP codon (which do not count in this calculation):	48 nu
All of exon Z is removed; there had been 142 nucleotides coding for amino acids in it:	142 nu
Total nucleotides removed:	387 nu

Dividing this by 3, we conclude that *your patient's β-spectrin is 129 amino acids shorter than that of a normal person.*

b. Your patient's β-spectrin has its C-terminal region deleted by this splicing error. The C-terminal region is where the β-spectrin is postulated to interact with α-spectrin to make a dimer. An abnormal spectrin dimer may not associate well with ankyrin and other elements of the erythrocyte cytoskeleton, and this could lead to unusual morphology of the erythrocytes. This would lead, in turn, to excess lysis of the erythrocytes, which would cause weakness because less oxygen would be delivered to the tissues.

Your patient has HEREDITARY ELLIPTOCYTOSIS.

References

Dhermy, D., Lecomte, M. C., Garbarz, M., Bournier, O., Galand, C., Gautero, H., Feo, C., Alloisio, N., Delaunay, J., and Boivin, P. Spectrin β-chain variant associated with hereditary elliptocytosis. *J. Clin. Invest.* 70: 707, 1982.

Gallagher, P. G., Tse, W. T., Costa, F., Scarpa, A., Boivin, P., Delaunay, J., and Forget, B. G. A splice site mutation of the β-spectrin gene causing exon skipping in hereditary elliptocytosis associated with a truncated β-spectrin. *J. Biol. Chem.* 266: 15154, 1991.

Lux, S. E., and Becker, P. S. Disorders of the red cell membrane skeleton: hereditary spherocytosis and hereditary elliptocytosis. C. R. Scriver, A. L. Beaudet, W. S. Sly, and D. Valle (Eds.). *The Metabolic Basis of Inherited Disease.* New York: McGraw-Hill, 1989, Vol. II, Chap. 95, p. 2367.

Tse, W. T., Lecomte, M.-C., Costa, F. F., Garbarz, M., Feo, C., Boivin, P., Dherym, D., Forget, B. G. Point mutation in the β-spectrin gene associated with αI/74 hereditary elliptocytosis. *J. Clin. Invest.* 86: 909, 1990.

Answer 65

a. Microtubule-associated proteins from a wide variety of sources can induce tubulin to polymerize into microtubules. It is not surprising that leukocyte tubulin can be made to assemble into microtubules by addition of brain microtubule-associated proteins. Although the best studied microtubule-associated proteins are those from mammalian brain, a number of such proteins have been identified in other tissues. Therefore, the likely defect in this patient might be in leukocyte microtubule-associated proteins.

b. Microtubules play major roles in the activity of leukocytes. They are necessary for chemotaxis. Interestingly, disruption of microtubules does not abolish random migration but will prevent directed migration in response to a stimulus. Microtubule assembly also appears to be necessary for pseudopod formation. Without directional motility, the leukocytes will not migrate to the lesion in the skin window test. Microtubules are also involved in secretion; if microtubule assembly is poor, the secretory granules will not be able to empty their contents and the granules will grow larger and denser.

References

Anderson, D. C., Smith, S. W., and Springer, T. A. Leukocyte adhesion deficiency and other disorders of leukocyte motility. C. R. Scriver, A. L. Beaudet, W. S. Sly, and D. Valle (Eds.). *The Metabolic Basis of Inherited Disease.* New York: McGraw-Hill, 1989, Vol. II, Chap. 113, p. 2751.

Gallin, J. I., Malech, H. L., Wright, D. G., Whisnant, J. K., and Kirkpatrick, C. H. Recurrent severe infections in a child with abnormal leukocyte function: possible relationship to increased microtubule assembly. *Blood* 51: 919, 1978.

Malech, H. L., Root, R. K., and Gallin, J. I. Structural analysis of human neutrophil migration. Centriole, microtubule, and microfilament orientation and function during chemotaxis. *J. Cell Biol.* 75: 666, 1977.

Oliver, J. M., Zurier, R. B., and Berlin, R. D. Concanavalin A cap formation on polymorphonuclear leukocytes of normal and beige (Chediak–Higashi) mice. *Nature* 253: 471, 1975.

White, J. G., and Clawson, C. C. The Chediak–Higashi syndrome: microtubules in monocytes and lymphocytes. *Am. J. Hematol.* 7: 439, 1979.

Answer 66

a. A normal leukocyte has various ways of destroying pathogenic bacteria. Arrival of the appropriate signal (such as a chemotactic factor) at the leukocyte membrane can trigger a respiratory burst in which O_2^-, H_2O_2, and HOCl are released into a phagocytic vacuole. It appears that the burst is defective in your patient's leukocytes. Probably some step in the pathway is defective. When the signal reaches the leukocyte, it catalyzes formation of inositol 1,4,5-trisphosphate, which in turn leads to an increase in intracellular calcium and to phosphorylation of certain proteins by protein kinase C. The defect is not likely to be at one of these steps since we are told that there is no change in inositol 1,4,5-trisphosphate or in phosphorylation of proteins. These initial changes turn on the NADPH oxidase, which catalyzes this reaction:

$$2O_2 + NADPH \rightarrow 2O_2^- + NADP^+ + H^+$$

Superoxide dismutase then converts the superoxide anion (O_2^-) into hydrogen peroxide:

$$2O_2^- + 2H^+ \rightarrow H_2O_2 + O_2$$

Myeloperoxidase converts H_2O_2 into hypochlorite (HOCl):

$$H_2O_2 + 2Cl^- \rightarrow 2HOCl$$

The fact that H_2O_2 is not being made means that the defect is in either NADPH oxidase or superoxide dismutase. Since $NADP^+$ is also low, the defective enzyme must be *NADPH oxidase*. NADPH oxidase is actually a complex of at least four polypeptide chains. Two of these, with molecular weights of 91 and 22 kD, constitute a cytochrome, called cytochrome b_{558} or cytochrome b_{-245}. The other two components are polypeptides of 47 and 67 kD. In addition to these components, there may be an NADPH-binding protein and a *ras*-like G-protein called *rap*. The cytochrome portion is a membrane protein and also binds to FAD. In NADPH oxidase, the electrons flow from NADPH to FAD to cytochrome b_{-245} to O_2. In a normal person, the cytochrome and *ras* are anchored in the membrane, while the other parts are free in solution. Upon stimulation, the 47-kD protein becomes phosphorylated and then catalyzes the association of all the other components to form the active NADPH complex.

It would appear that the defective protein is the 91-kD subunit of the cytochrome. The defect is as follows:

Codon number:	414	415	416
Your patient:			
DNA:	ACA	CAC	TTC
RNA:	ACA	CAC	UUC
Protein:	Thr	His	Phe
Normal person:			
DNA:	ACA	CCC	TTC
RNA:	ACA	CCC	UUC
Protein:	Thr	Pro	Phe

Your patient has a histidine at position 415 of the large subunit of his cytochrome b_{558} instead of a proline. One could readily imagine that the disappearance of a proline could cause an extension of an α helix and otherwise disrupt the tertiary or secondary structure of the whole complex. The change could not be too drastic because the components which are supposed to get phosphorylated still do so. It is possible that the mutation alters the interaction of subunits within the NADPH oxidase in such a fashion that the reaction could not take place.

b. O_2^- leads to formation of hypochlorite and free radicals, such as OH·, which are toxic to bacteria. It is not exactly clear how these hurt bacteria, but it is possible that they disrupt electron transport in bacteria or oxidize important iron-sulfur centers.

Your patient has CHRONIC GRANULOMATOUS DISEASE. It is interesting and perhaps hopeful that gene therapy is being attempted to treat this disease and is so far giving promising results.

References

Dinauer, M. C., Curnutte, J. T., Rosen, H., and Orkin, S. H. A missense mutation in the neutrophil cytochrome b heavy chain in cytochrome-positive X-linked chronic granulomatous disease. *J. Clin. Invest.* 84: 2012, 1989.

Forehand, J. R., Nauseef, W. N., and Johnston, R. B. Inherited disorders of phagocyte killing. C. R. Scriver, A. L. Beaudet, W. S. Sly, and D. Valle (Eds.). *The Metabolic Basis of Inherited Disease.* New York: McGraw-Hill, 1989, Vol. II, Chap. 114, p. 2779.

Porter, C. D., Parkar, M. H., Levinsky, R. J., Collins, M. K. L., and Kinnon, C. X-linked chronic granulomatous disease: correction of NADPH oxidase defect by retrovirus-mediated expression of gp91-*phox. Blood* 82: 2196, 1993.

Smith, R. M., and Curnutte, J. T. Molecular basis of chronic granulomatous disease. *Blood* 77: 673, 1991.

Answer 67

a. When phagocytic leukocytes are stimulated appropriately (as by a chemotactic peptide), they have a respiratory burst, whose last step is the production of hypochlorite from H_2O_2, catalyzed by myeloperoxidase. The events of this burst are described in more detail in the answer to Problem 66. Since H_2O_2 is still produced by your patient's leukocytes, the defect must be in the step in which H_2O_2 is converted into hypochlorite, and therefore *myeloperoxidase,* which catalyzes this reaction, is likely to be the defective enzyme. Here is the myeloperoxidase reaction:

$$H_2O_2 + 2Cl^- \rightarrow 2HOCl$$

b. Hypochlorite is toxic to certain microorganisms, particularly *Candida.*

Reference

Forehand, J. R., Nauseef, W. N., and Johnston, R. B. Inherited disorders of phagocyte killing. C. R. Scriver, A. L. Beaudet, W. S. Sly, and D. Valle (Eds.). *The Metabolic Basis of Inherited Disease.* New York: McGraw-Hill, 1989, Vol. II, Chap. 114, p. 2779.

Answer 68

a. To do their job, leukocytes have to be able to adhere to pathogenic organisms as a first step toward destroying them. The glycoprotein β (called CD18 by the World Health Organization) (MW 95,000) is a component of three different complexes involved in adhesion. These complexes are Mac-1 (with the 170,000 MW αM protein), p150,95 (with the 150,000 MW αX protein), and LFA-1 (with the 177,000 MW αL protein). Mac-1, found in a variety of leukocytes, is the receptor for the complement component iC3b. It can also bind to endothelial cells. p150,95 has a cellular distribution similar to that of Mac-1 and appears to have the same binding characteristics. LFA-1 is found primarily in lymphocytes and monocytes (but not macrophages); it is involved in the T-cell-mediated responses. If these protein complexes are missing, the leukocytes will be unable to bind to bacteria which have been attacked by the complement system and which have iC3b on their surfaces.

b. You would expect these leukocytes to adhere to dead bacteria bound to C3b because αL is part of LFA-1, which is *not* a C3b receptor.

Reference
Forehand, J. R., Nauseef, W. N., and Johnston, R. B. Inherited disorders of phagocyte killing. C. R. Scriver, A. L. Beaudet, W. S. Sly, and D. Valle (Eds.). *The Metabolic Basis of Inherited Disease.* New York: McGraw-Hill, 1989, Vol. II, Chap. 114, p. 2779.

CHAPTER 10

The Immune System

Problem 69

Your patient is often getting infections, specifically bacterial infections caused by *Streptococcus*, *Pneumococcus*, *Meningococcus*, and *Hemophilus*. His immunoglobulin levels are normal, as are his levels of the classical complement proteins C1, C2, C4, C5, C6, C7, C8, and C9. His level of C3 is low, but the C3 he has is not altered; there is simply less of it. As an experiment, you draw some of your patient's blood and add some radioactive C3 to it. You find that it gets broken down to C3b much faster in your patient's blood than if you had added it to a normal person's blood. You check the levels of some of the alternative complement pathway components. You find that factors B, D, and H and properdin are normal.

a. Which protein is likely to be defective in your patient?

b. How does that cause the problems?

c. Write out the alternative pathway of complement.

Problem 70

Your patient is a 10-year-old girl with frequent attacks in which she experiences edematous swellings of her lips, pharynx, or tongue. She often complains of abdominal cramps. In a recent attack, she had laryngeal edema in which her voice became hoarse and then she became unable to breathe and an emergency tracheotomy had to be performed to save her life. You draw some blood and measure the levels of the complement components. C1, C2, C3, C4, C5, C6, C7, C8, and C9; factors B, D, H, and I; and properdin are present at their normal levels. You do an experiment in which you mix the following components: (1) sheep erythrocyte membranes, (2) IgG specific for sheep erythrocyte membranes, (3) C1, (4) C2, (5) C3, and (6) C4. To this mixture you add either your patient's serum or a normal person's serum (from each of which C1, C2, C3, C4, and factors B and D have been removed by immunoaffinity chromatography). You measure the production of C3b and find that much more C3b is produced in your patient's serum than in that of a normal person. You now examine the rate at which C2 and C4 get cleaved and find that it is much higher in your patient's serum than in a normal person's serum.

    a. What protein is deficient in your patient?

    b. What does that protein do?

    c. What would you predict would happen if you injected C1s̄ subcutaneously into a normal person?

Problem 71

Your patient has a disease in which at night, his urine turns red. You analyze the red pigment and find that it is hemoglobin. You analyze the complement proteins in his blood and find that they appear normal. You then do an experiment in which you add C5b, C6, C7, C8, and C9 from a normal person to erythrocytes from your patient and from a normal person. You find that his erythrocytes lyse more quickly than do those of a normal person in the same experiment. You then measure the ability of the individual components of complement to bind to membranes purified from your patient's erythrocytes and to those of a normal person. You find no difference except that C8 binds to the erythrocytes of a normal person but not to those of your patient.

a. What protein is missing in your patient? Do not worry about getting the right name for it; just say what it does.

b. How does its absence induce the symptoms?

Note: This disease may have multiple causes. You are dealing with only one of them in this problem.

Problem 72

Your patient has a disease in which at night when he is ill, his urine turns red. You analyze the red pigment and find that it is hemoglobin. You find that his erythrocyte membranes lack decay-accelerating factor. You culture some of his cell lines and then lyse them. To the lysates you add radioactive UDP-N-acetylglucosamine. You find that synthesis of radioactive glycolipids was much less than normal.

a. What is missing from your patient's decay-accelerating factor? Draw the missing structure.

b. How is this structure made? Which step is defective in your patient?

c. What is the role of decay-accelerating factor? How does its defect explain the symptoms?

Problem 73

Your patient is subject to repeated infections and has previously received a diagnosis of systemic lupus erythematosus. You analyze a sample of his blood for the complement proteins, using an ELISA technique, and find that he appears to be missing C2. In this ELISA you use a monoclonal antibody that recognizes both the activated and the inactive form of C2. You culture some of his fibroblasts and extract the mRNA coding for C2. Using appropriate oligonucleotides and the PCR reaction, you are able to obtain a cDNA. The following is a portion of the sequence of the cDNA compared to that which you would find for a normal person:

Your patient: ACAAAGGATCTTgAGCTTTGAGATC
Normal person: ACAAAGGAAAGCCTGGGCCGT. . . ATCTTCAGCTTTGAGATC
                7   8
                0   5
                9   0

Assume that the first nucleotide in the sequence marks the beginning of a codon. In the normal person's sequence ". . ." means a long section of cDNA whose sequence is not given here. The number of the position in the sequence of a normal person is given.

a. What was the mutational event that occurred in your patient?

b. During complement activation, C2 is cleaved by C1s̄. Knowing that C1s̄ resembles trypsin in its sequence, which position in the sequence of C2 in a normal person (shown above) corresponds to the site in C2 where C1s̄ cleaves?

c. Why does your patient appear to have no C2 by the ELISA test?

Problem 74

Your patient has suffered severe recurring bacterial infections, particularly pneumonia and meningitis. Two of his mother's brothers died before the age of 6, apparently with the same ailment. Analysis of your patient's blood shows that he lacks IgG and, in fact, lacks B cells. You do a bone marrow biopsy and examine the pre-B cells. You find a gene that is altered in your patient; the gene codes for a protein-tyrosine kinase of the *src* family. Here are the sequences in the vicinity of the mutation:

Your patient: GACGTGGCCATCGAGATGATGAAAGAAGGC
Normal person: GACGTGGCCATCAAGATGATCAAAGAAGGC

In searching the literature on *src* proteins, you find a paper that reports that *p*-fluorosulfonylbenzoyl 5'-adenosine, an affinity analog of ATP, when reacted with lysine 295 of another *src* protein can completely inactivate the protein-tyrosine kinase activity. The partial amino acid sequence of the other *src* protein is:

Codon number:	291	292	293	294	295	296	297	298	299	300
Amino acid:	His	Val	Ala	Ilu	Lys	Thr	Leu	Lys	Pro	Gly

a. How might the observed mutation alter the activity of the enzyme?

b. In very general terms, try to connect a mutation in this type of protein with your patient's lack of B cells.

Problem 75

Your patient has suffered severe recurring bacterial infections, particularly pneumonia and meningitis. Two of his mother's brothers died before the age of 6, apparently with the same ailment. Analysis of your patient's blood shows that he lacks IgG and, in fact, lacks B cells. You do a bone marrow biopsy and examine the pre-B cells. You find a gene that is altered in your patient; the gene codes for a protein-tyrosine kinase of the *src* family. Here are the sequences in the vicinity of the mutation:

Your patient: CGAGACCTGGCAGCTCAAAACTGTTTGGTAAAC
Normal person: CGAGACCTGGCAGCTCGAAACTGTTTGGTAAAC

You compare the sequences of all known protein kinases. You find that certain regions on all protein kinases have very similar sequences; an example is the region where ATP binds. You also find one region in the sequences of protein kinases that appears to be distinctly different for protein kinases which phosphorylate serine or threonine and for protein kinases which phosphorylate tyrosine residues. The differences are shown here. For each type of kinase, the top line represents the most common sequence; substitutions that occur occasionally are shown underneath.

1. Ser/Thr kinases

              Asp-Leu- Lys-Pro-Glu-Asn
                 Val   Leu Gln
                 Ilu   Ilu Asp
                Met   Asp Asn
                           Thr His
                           Ser Thr
                             Ala

Consensus: Asp-X-Lys-X-X-Asn

2. Tyrosine kinases

              Asp-Leu-Ala-Ala-Arg-Asn
                Val Arg Ser Ala
                       Cys
                       Thr

Consensus: Asp-L/V-Ala-X-Arg-Asn   *or*   Asp-Leu-Arg-X-Ala-Asn
[L = Leu; V = Val]

    a. How might the observed mutation alter the activity of enzyme?

    b. How might such an alteration give rise to the observed symptoms?

Problem 76

Your patient has just died at age 39. Autopsy results show extensive proteinaceous deposits in his viscera. You analyze the protein deposits and find that they react with an antibody to human lysozyme. Your identification of the protein as lysozyme is confirmed by sequencing. The sequence shows a difference in one area, however. Here are the partial sequences:

Residue number:	50	51	52	53	54	55	56	57	58	59	60
Your patient:	Arg	Ser	Thr	Asp	Tyr	Gly	Thr	Phe	Gln	Ile	Asn
Normal person:	Arg	Ser	Thr	Asp	Tyr	Gly	Ile	Phe	Gln	Ile	Asn

Your reading of the literature has revealed a great many lysozyme sequences among the vertebrates. At position 56, all of them have either isoleucine, leucine, or valine. A scientist substituted a valine at position 56 in chicken egg white lysozyme by site-directed mutagenesis and showed no difference in activity. X-ray crystallography of normal human lysozyme shows that isoleucine 56 and serine 36 are juxtaposed (Figure P76-1).

a. What is the function of lysozyme?

b. Speculate on the probable effect of substituting a threonine at position 56. How might this lead to disease?

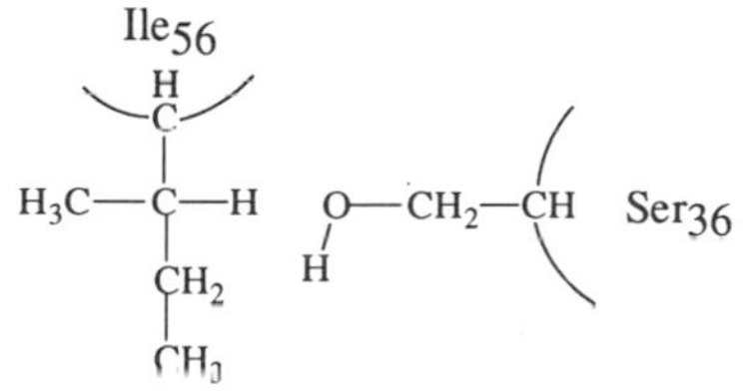

FIGURE P76-1. **Arrangement of ile^{56} and ser^{36} in lysozyme.**

Problem 77

Your patient has frequent bacterial infections. His serum levels of IgG, IgA, and IgE are decreased, while his levels of IgM are greatly increased, compared to those for a normal person. You purify his B cells and T cells and find that they have a decreased ability to interact. You obtain purified CD40 protein from B cells and measure its ability to bind to the T cells. This is greatly decreased for your patient. After many experiments, you obtain a protein (protein X) that is normally expressed on the membranes of T cells. You find that this protein is present in greatly diminished quantities in your patient. You sequence the gene for protein X and find the following:

Codon number:	35	36	37
Your patient:	GAC	AGG	TTA
Normal person:	GAC	ATG	TTA

a. What is the likely role of protein X?

b. What is the defect in your patient's protein X?

c. Why might this defect result in the observed symptoms?

Answer 69

a. Your patient does not appear to have a mutation in his C3, but it does seem to be getting broken down faster than would be the case with a normal person. Normally, C3 is cleaved by C4b2a in the classical pathway and by C3 convertase in the alternative pathway. The classical pathway generally starts with an antigen, whereas the alternative pathway is constantly getting under way and generating small amounts of C3b. The classical pathway is unlikely to be the problem here, since an overactive C4b2a complex is unlikely to increase susceptibility to disease. Hence it is more probable that the problem is that C3 convertase is too active. C3 convertase is formed from C3, factor B, and factor D. C3 convertase cleaves C3 into C3b and C3a. The C3b could then bind to the surface of certain susceptible pathogens. If no antigen is available, C3b and C3 convertase will be degraded by factors H and I. A likely cause of your patient's problem is a defect in either factor H or factor I. This would increase activity of C3 convertase and more C3 would be degraded. Defects in factor I are more common than defects in factor H. Also, factor I is a proteolytic enzyme (a serine protease) whereas factor H is more likely to act noncovalently in facilitating the interaction of C3 convertase with factor I.

b. Without factor I, C3 gets broken down, since factor I inhibits C3 convertase. Lowering C3 inhibits the alternative and classical pathways, which greatly increases the likelihood of infection.

c. The alternative pathway of complement is summarized as follows:

$$C3 + H_2O \rightarrow C3 - H_2O$$
$$C3 - H_2O + B + D \rightarrow C3 \text{ convertase}$$
$$C3 \text{ convertase} + C3 \rightarrow C3b + C3a$$
$$C3b + B + D \rightarrow C3b + Bb + Ba + D$$
$$C3b + Bb \rightarrow C3b, Bb$$
$$C3b, Bb \rightarrow C3b_n, Bb \rightarrow C3b_n, P, Bb$$
$$C3b_n, P, Bb + C5 \rightarrow C5a + C5b$$
$$C5b + C6 + C7 + C8 + 6\ C9 \rightarrow \text{membrane attack complex}$$

Reference

Winkelstein, J. A., and Colten, H. R. Genetically determined disorders of the complement system. C. R. Scriver, A. L. Beaudet, W. S. Sly, and D. Valle (Eds.). *The Metabolic Basis of Inherited Disease*. New York: McGraw-Hill, 1989, Vol. II, Chap. 111, p. 2711.

Answer 70

a. All the complement factors are present in normal amounts. Hence it is unlikely that there is overproduction of one of those proteins. In your experiment you look at the beginning of the classical complement pathway. You mix an antigen (sheep erythrocyte membranes) with the corresponding antibody and the complement components C1, C2, C3, and C4, together with serum, and you find that C3b production is much greater than normal. C3b is produced by the action of C3 convertase (which contains factors B and D) and by the C4b2a complex. Since your experimental system lacks B and D, then, obviously, there can be no C3 convertase here. Therefore, there must be more C4b2a complex in your patient's sample. The C4b2a complex is formed from C4b and C2a, which are in turn produced by cleavage of C4 and C2. If there is more C4b2a complex, there is likely to be excess cleavage of C4 and C2. These cleavages are carried out by the C1 complex, specifically by the activated protease C1s̄. If there is excess cleavage, the cause cannot be an abnormality in C1s̄, because you used exogenous C1 in the experiment and still got excess cleavage of C4 and C2. By the same argument, C2 and C4 cannot be altered in some way so as to be more susceptible to being cleaved. Thus there has to be something in your patient's serum, other than the above-mentioned factors, which increases the activity of C1s̄. Your patient, therefore, lacks *C1 inhibitor*, a 105-kD glycoprotein with a sequence that appears to place it in the family of serine protease inhibitors.

b. C1 inhibitor inactivates C1s̄, the active form of C1s, a component of the C1 complex. By inhibiting C1s̄, C1 inhibitor can slow down the cleavage of C4 and C2. Since your patient has a deficiency in C1 inhibitor, he will have excessive cleavage of C4 and C2, excess formation of the C4b2a complex, and excessive production of C3b.

c. Since a major factor in the disease caused by C1 inhibitor deficiency is the excessive production of C1s̄, one could argue that injection of C1s̄ into a person would lead to at least localized edema, and this has been observed. The actual mechanism by which C1 inhibitor deficiency results in edema is not known.

Your patient has HEREDITARY ANGIOEDEMA.

Reference

Winkelstein, J. A., and Colten, H. R. Genetically determined disorders of the complement system. C. R. Scriver, A. L. Beaudet, W. S. Sly, and D. Valle (Eds.). *The Metabolic Basis of Inherited Disease.* New York: McGraw-Hill, 1989, Vol. II, Chap. 111, p. 2711.

Answer 71

a. The components C5b, C6, C7, C8, and C9 constitute the membrane attack complex (MAC) of complement, the complex that causes lysis of the target cell. The fact that mixing these components causes increased lysis in your patient's cells compared to those of a normal person implies that the MAC is somehow more active with your patient's erythrocytes than with those of a normal person. Since these are presumably exogenous complement factors which you are adding, they could not be altered in your patient; hence the alteration in your patient is likely to be in some factor that regulates (i.e., inhibits) the MAC. There are a variety of such factors that could be present on the erythrocytes. The fact that C8 does not bind to membrane proteins from your patient's erythrocytes but does bind to those of a normal person implies that your patient is lacking a protein that is specific for C8. This protein is called C8 *binding protein* or C8 *inhibiting protein* or *homologous restriction factor.*

b. The role of this protein is not to inhibit the activity of MAC when it is doing its normal function, such as lysing a pathogenic bacterium, but rather to protect the erythrocyte from attack by MACs. Although most of the MACs will bind to the bacteria that are infecting your patient, the extras will bind to the nearest surface, which is likely to be that of the erythrocyte. If these MACs do not encounter the C8 binding protein, they will proceed to lyse the erythrocyte and cause it to release its hemoglobin into the blood.

Your patient has PAROXYSMAL NOCTURNAL HEMOGLOBINURIA.

References

Hänsch, G. M. The homologous species restriction of the complement attack: structure and function of the C8 binding protein. *Curr. Topics Microbiol. Immunol.* 140. 108, 1988.

Hänsch, G. M., Schönermark, S., and Roelcke, D. Paroxysmal nocturnal hemoglobinuria type III: lack of an erythrocyte membrane protein restricting the lysis by C5b-9. *J. Clin. Invest.* 80: 7, 1987.

Schultz, D. R. Erythrocyte membrane protein deficiencies in paroxysmal nocturnal hemoglobinuria. *Am. J. Med.* 87: 3-22N, 1989.

Zalman, L. S. Homologous restriction factor. *Curr. Topics Microbiol. Immunol.* 178: 87, 1992.

Answer 72

a. A patient whose urine becomes red is likely to have hemoglobin in his urine, which in turn suggests abnormal lysis of his erythrocytes. Decay-accelerating factor (DAF) is a protein that is anchored to the erythrocyte membrane via a glycophosphatidylinositol (GPI) anchor (Figure A72-1). If the anchor is missing, the decay-accelerating factor will be missing from the membranes. The fact that your patient's cells cannot convert UDP-*N*-acetylglucosamine into glycolipid suggests that the biosynthesis of the glycophosphatidylinositol anchor is defective.

You will notice that there are three fatty acid moieties in the anchor. Two of them are part of the phosphatidyl inositol; the third is attached directly to the inositol at some as yet undetermined position. The function

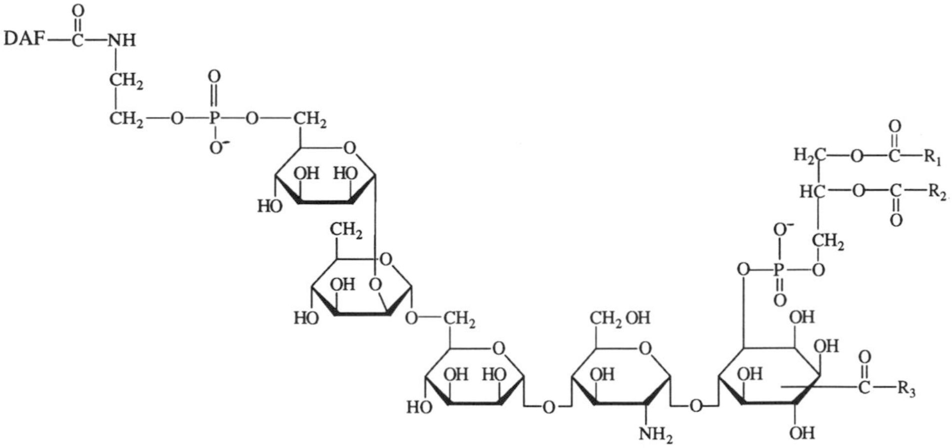

FIGURE A72-1. **Structure of glycophosphatidylinositol. It is not known precisely where the fatty acid attaches to the inositol residue.**

of the third fatty acid is not clear. Some other GPI anchors do not contain this third fatty acid. One possibility is that the third fatty acid may have a regulatory role. Normally, phospholipase C can cleave between the ethanolamine and the phosphate, thereby releasing the bound protein. However, if the third fatty acid is present, the anchor cannot be removed by phospholipase C; a second enzyme, called deacylase, is necessary to remove the fatty acid so that phospholipase C can act.

b. The pathway for synthesizing glycophosphatidylinositol is shown in Figure A72-2. The first step in the pathway involves the transfer of N-acetylglucosamine from UDP onto phosphatidylinositol to make a glycolipid. This step is defective in your patient. In the final step, the C-terminal 28 residues of DAF are removed, making Ser^{319} the new C-terminal and the glycophosphatidylinositol is attached to that serine. The signal for reaction with the glycophosphatidylinositol is the presence of the 17-amino acid hydrophobic peptide (residues 331 to 347) and the presence of two small amino acids (Ser^{319} and Gly^{320}) at the cleavage/attachment site.

c. Decay-accelerating factor (DAF) is situated on the external membranes of erythrocytes. It can bind to any fragments of C3b or C4b that inadvertently attach themselves to the membrane. By binding to them, DAF inhibits them from forming C3 convertase complexes, whose action could lead to the lysis of the erythrocyte. As few as 70 molecules of DAF bound to an erythrocyte can completely prevent assembly of the C4b2a complex, which cleaves C3 to generate C3a and C3b. The C3b fragment can bind to the nearest membrane and mediate immune adherence, in which certain leukocytes bind to the C3b and destroy the cell to whose membrane the C3b is bound. The C3b fragment can also join with the C4b2a complex to generate a C5 convertase; this complex cleaves C5 to generate C5a and C5b. C5b joins with C6, C7, C8, and C9 to form the membrane-attack complex, which can lyse the target cell. Under normal circumstances the C4b2a and membrane-attack complexes will bind to the original target cell, generally a pathogen recognized by an antibody. However, the large number of erythrocytes in the blood creates the possibility that a C4b or C2a may drift away from its point of origin and bind to an erythrocyte membrane. Since the complement proteins are essentially mindless agents of destruction, the results of such inadvertent binding could be the lysis of the erythrocyte. That is the reason for

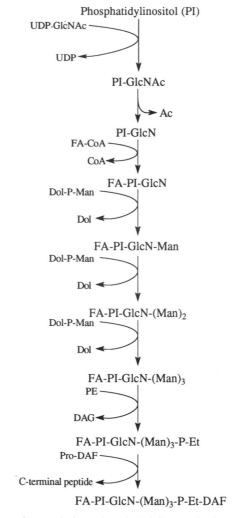

FIGURE A72-2. **Biosynthesis of glycophosphatidylinositol. The step in which the acetyl group is removed is stimulated by GTP hydrolysis. Abbreviations: Ac, acetyl; DAF, decay-accelerating factor; DAG, diacylglycerol; Dol, dolichol; Et, ethanolamine; FA, fatty acyl; GlcN, glucosamine; GlcNAc, *N*-acetylglucosamine; M, mannose; P, phosphate; PE, phosphatidylethanolamine; PI, phosphatidylinositol. Some details of the pathway are not certain.**

DAF; it is normally present on erythrocyte membranes and will prevent formation of any C4b2a complexes and hence protect the erythrocyte from destruction. Your patient lacks DAF; therefore, he does not have this protection. When he is ill and his immune system is generating larger amounts of activated complement proteins, some of them will attach to his erythrocytes and bring about their lysis. This is why his urine turns red when he is ill. Why this should happen primarily at night is not clear.

Your patient has PAROXYSMAL NOCTURNAL HEMOGLO-BINURIA.

References

Armstrong, C., Schubert, J., Ueda, E., Knez, K. K., Gelperin, D., Hirose, S., Silber, R., Hollan, S., Schmidt, R. E., and Medof, M. E. Affected paroxysmal nocturnal hemoglobinuria T lymphocytes harbor a common defect in assembly of N-acetyl-D-glucosamine inositol phospholipid corresponding to that in class A thy-1⁻ murine lymphoma mutants. J. Biol. Chem. 267: 25347, 1992.

Davitz, M. A. Decay accelerating factor (DAF): a review of its function and structure. Acta Med Scand., Suppl. 715: 111, 1987.

Doering, T. L., Masterson, W. J., Hart, G. W., and Englund, P. T. Biosynthesis of glycosyl phosphatidylinositol membrane anchors. J. Biol. Chem. 265: 611, 1990.

Englund, P. T. The structure and biosynthesis of glycosyl phosphatidylinositol protein anchors. Annu. Rev. Biochem. 62: 121, 1993.

Hillmen, P., Bessler, M., Mason, M. J., Watkins, W. M., and Luzzatto, L. Specific defect in N-acetylglucosamine incorporation in the biosynthesis of the glycosylphosphatidylinositol anchor in cloned cell lines from patients with paroxysmal nocturnal hemoglobinuria. Proc. Natl. Acad. Sci. USA 90: 5272, 1993.

Hirose, S., Prince, G. M., Sevlever, D., Ravi, L., Rosenberry, T. L., Ueda, E., and Medof, M. E. Characterization of putative glycoinositol phospholipid anchor precursors in mammalian cells. Localization of phosphoethanolamine. J. Biol. Chem. 267: 16968, 1992.

Kamitani, T., Menon, A. K., Hallaq, Y., Warren, C. D., and Yeh, E. T. H. Complexity of ethanolamine phosphate addition in the biosynthesis of glycosylphosphatidylinositol anchors in mammalian cells. J. Biol. Chem. 267: 24611, 1992.

McConville, M. J., and Ferguson, M. A. J. The structure, biosynthesis and function of glycosylated phosphatidylinositols in the parasitic protozoa and higher eukaryotes. Biochem. J. 294: 305, 1993.

Moran, P., and Caras, I. W. A nonfunctional sequence converted to a signal for glyco-phosphatidylinositol membrane anchor attachment. J. Cell Biol. 115: 329, 1991

Moran, P., Raab, H., Kohr, W. J., and Caras, I. W. Glycophospholipid membrane anchor attachment. Molecular analysis of the cleavage/attachment site. *J. Biol. Chem.* 266: 1250, 1991.

Puoti, A., and Conzelmann, A. Characterization of abnormal free glycophosphatidylinositols accumulating in mutant lymphoma cells of classes B, E, F, and H. *J. Biol. Chem.* 268: 7215, 1993.

Stevens, V. L. Regulation of glycosylphosphatidylinositol biosynthesis by GTP. Stimulation of N-acetylglucosamine-phosphatidylinositol deacetylation. *J. Biol. Chem.* 268: 9718, 1993.

Takahashi, M., Takeda, J., Hirose, S., Hyman, R., Inoue, N., Miyata, T., Ueda, E., Kitani, T., Medof, M. E., and Kinoshita, T. Deficient biosynthesis of N-acetylglucosaminyl-phosphatidylinositol, the first intermediate of glycosyl phosphatidylinositol anchor biosynthesis, in cell lines established from patients with paroxysmal nocturnal hemoglobinuria. *J. Exp. Med.* 177: 517, 1993.

Takeda, J., Miyata, T., Kawagoe, K., Iida, Y., Endo, Y., Fujita, T., Takahashi, M., Kitani, T., and Kinoshita, T. Deficiency of the GPI anchor caused by a somatic mutation of the PIG-A gene in paroxysmal nocturnal hemoglobinuria. *Cell* 73: 703, 1993.

Tartakoff, A. M., and Singh, N. How to make a glycoinositol phospholipid anchor. *Trends Biochem. Sci.* 17: 470, 1992.

Answer 73

a. By lining up the nucleotides appropriately, it appears that there has been a deletion of nucleotides 717 to 850 (or 716 to 849):

Your patient:	ACAAAGGA	TCTTCAGCTTTGAGATC
Normal person:	ACAAAGGAAAGCCTGGGCCGT. . . ATCTTCAGCTTTGAGATC	
	7	8
	0	5
	9	0

b. You have to convert the nucleotide sequence into RNA and then into the protein sequence as follows:

DNA:	ACA	AAG	GAA	AGC	CTG	GGC	CGT
RNA:	ACA	AAG	GAA	AGC	CUG	GGC	CGU
Protein:	Thr	Lys	Glu	Ser	Leu	Gly	Arg

C1s will cleave after lysine. On the nucleotide sequence that corresponds to between positions 714 and 715.

c. Let's look at your patient's sequence:

DNA: ACA AAG GAT CTT CAG CTT TGA GAT C
RNA: ACA AAG GAU CUU CAG CUU UGA GAU C
Protein: Thr Lys Glu Leu Gln Leu STOP

The result of the deletion of either 133 or 134 base pairs (a number that is not divisible by 3) is a frameshift causing a new reading of the amino acids and resulting in a stop codon being generated. There is more to it, however, because the active portion of C2 is that which occurs after the C1s cleavage point. Your patient would end up with an "activated" C2 molecule that is four amino acids long (Glu-Leu-Gln-Leu). This would be inactive and not show up in an ELISA, since the antibody used in this ELISA is to the activated form of C2. (This is a monoclonal antibody; therefore, all its molecules have the same specificity. Since it recognizes both the activated form of C2 as well as the inactive precursor, its epitope must be in the region of C2 corresponding to the active enzyme and this region is on the C-terminal side of where C1s cleaves C2.) Its epitope would almost certainly have been in the deleted portion of the protein.

Your patient has TYPE I COMPLEMENT C2 DEFICIENCY.

Reference

Johnson, C. A., Densen, P., Hurford, R. K., Colten, H. R., and Wetsel, R. A. Type I human complement C2 deficiency: a 28-base pair gene deletion causes skipping of exon 6 during RNA splicing. *J. Biol. Chem.* 267: 9347, 1992.

Answer 74

a. The protein sequence in the vicinity of the mutation can be predicted as follows:

Your patient:
  DNA: GAC GTG GCC ATC GAG ATG ATC AAA GAA GGC
  RNA: GAC GUG GCC AUC GAG AUG AUC AAA GAA GGC
  Protein: Asp Val Ala Ilu Glu Met Ilu Lys Glu Gly
Normal person:
  DNA: GAC GTG GCC ATC AAG ATG ATC AAA GAA GGC
  RNA: GAC GUG GCC AUC AAG AUG AUC AAA GAA GGC
  Protein: Asp Val Ala Ilu Lys Met Ilu Lys Glu Gly

Comparing the sequence of this protein from a normal person with the sequence of the other *src* protein (p60^{src}) shows that we are clearly looking at the corresponding portions of the sequence:

| Normal sequence: | Asp Val Ala Ilu Lys Met Ilu Lys Glu Gly |
| *src* protein: | His Val Ala Ilu Lys Thr Leu Lys Pro Gly |

The experiment with the other *src* protein indicates that ATP must bind at or very close to Lys^{295}. Comparison of the sequences shows that the altered amino acid in your patient's protein is in an equivalent region of the sequence as Lys^{295}. Therefore, it is likely that the mutated enzyme is inactive by being unable to bind to ATP.

b. Protein kinases of the *src* type are often involved in development and differentiation. An inactive protein could mess up development and result in inability of pre-B cells to turn into B cells.

Your patient has X-LINKED AGAMMAGLOBULINEMIA.

References

Kamps. M. P., Taylor, S. S., and Sefton, B. M. Direct evidence that oncogenic tyrosine kinases and cyclic AMP-dependent protein kinase have homologous ATP-binding sites. *Nature* 310: 589, 1984.

Vetrie, D., Vorechovský, I., Sideras, P., Holland, J., Davies, A., Flinter, F., Hammarström, L., Kinnon, C., Levinsky, R., Bobrow, M., Smith, C. I. E., and Bentley, D. R. The gene involved in X-linked agammaglobulinaemia is a member of the *src* family of protein-tyrosine kinases. *Nature* 361: 226, 1993.

Answer 75

a. Look at the protein sequence in the region of the mutation you have discovered.

Your patient:	
DNA:	CGA GAC CTG GCA GCT CAA AAC TGT TTG GTA AAC
RNA:	CGA GAC CUG GCA GCU CAA AAC UGU UUG GUA AAC
Protein:	Arg Asp Leu Ala Ala Gln Asn Cys Leu Val Asn

Normal person:

DNA:	CGA GAC CTG GCA GCT CGA AAC TGT TTG GTA AAC
RNA:	CGA GAC CUG GCA GCU CGA AAC UGU UUG GUA AAC
Protein:	Arg Asp Leu Ala Ala Arg Asn Cys Leu Val Asn

Compare the sequence in a normal person with that of the sequences of serine/threonine-directed kinases and tyrosine-directed kinases:

Normal person:	Arg Asp Leu Ala Ala Arg Asn Cys Leu Val Asn
Tyr kinase:	Asp-L/V- Ala- X- Arg- Asn
Tyr kinase:	Asp-Leu- Arg- X- Ala- Asn
Ser/thr kinase:	Asp-Leu- Lys- Pro- Glu- Asn

The mutation is clearly in a region that distinguishes serine/threonine protein kinases from tyrosine protein kinases. If you did not already know this, you would conclude that your protein is a tyrosine kinase rather than a serine/threonine kinase, because of the sequence similarities. This region is probably where the substrate binds. Alteration in substrate binding could inactivate the enzyme. The Arg → Gln mutation is one that does not occur in any known kinase at that position, which is either arginine, alanine, or glutamate. Interestingly, in tyrosine kinases the segment between the aspartate and the asparagine seems to require having an arginine somewhere between the two. Your patient's protein has no arginine in that region at all. It is not surprising that your patient's protein is not functional.

b. Protein kinases of the *src* type are often involved in development and differentiation. An inactive protein could mess up development and result in inability of pre-B cells to turn into B cells.

Your patient has X-LINKED AGAMMAGLOBULINEMIA.

References

Hanks, S. K., Quinn, A. M., and Hunter, T. The protein kinase family: conserved features and deduced phylogeny of the catalytic domains. *Science* 241: 42, 1988.

Vetrie, D., Vorechovský, I., Sideras, P., Holland, J., Davies, A., Flinter, F., Hammarström, L., Kinnon, C., Levinsky, R., Bobrow, M., Smith, C. I. E., and Bentley, D. R. The gene involved in the X-linked agammaglobulinaemia is a member of the *src* family of protein-tyrosine kinases. *Nature* 361: 226, 1993.

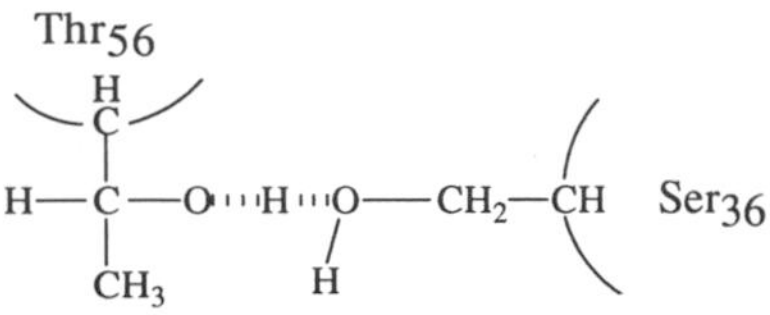

FIGURE A76-1. **Possible hydrogen bond in mutant lysozyme.**

Answer 76

a. Lysozyme cleaves the polysaccharides of certain bacterial cell walls. This makes the bacteria vulnerable to lysis. Hence lysozyme protects us from certain types of bacteria.

b. All normal lysozymes have either isoleucine, leucine, or valine at this position. Apparently, this position is supposed to be occupied by a hydrophobic amino acid of a certain size range. Clearly, threonine causes a problem, yet it is roughly in the same size range. Thus it is probably not the size of threonine that is the problem, but rather the fact that it has a hydroxyl group. If you substitute threonine into Figure P76-1, you will have a very probable hydrogen bond between Thr[56] and Ser[36] (Figure A76-1). The hatched lines indicate the hydrogen bond. The resulting stabilized structure of the protein may prolong its lifetime or simply allow it to polymerize more readily and cause the disease.

Your patient has HEREDITARY NONNEUROPATHIC SYSTEMIC AMYLOIDOSIS (OSTERTAG TYPE).

Reference

Pepys, M. B., Hawkins, P. N., Booth, D. R., Vigushin, D. M., Tennent, G. A., Soutar, A. K., Totty, N., Nhuyen, O., Blake, C. C. F., Terry, C. J., Feest, T. G., Zalin, A. M., and Hsuan, J. J. Human lysozyme gene mutations cause hereditary systemic amyloidosis. *Nature* 362: 553, 1993.

Answer 77

a. Protein X is the receptor for CD40. It allows the T cells to activate the B cells. Protein X is a 33-kD protein that has been given the name of TRAP (TNF-related activation protein). It is likely that when TRAP, which is on the T-cell membrane, binds to CD40, which is on the B-cell membrane, the B cell is induced to switch over to making immuno-globulins other than IgM.

b. First, the altered residue is identified.

Codon number:	35	36	37
Your patient:			
DNA:	CAG	AGG	ATT
RNA:	CAG	AGG	AUU
Protein:	Gln	Arg	Ilu
Normal person:			
DNA:	CAG	ATG	ATT
RNA:	CAG	AUG	AUU
Protein:	Gln	Met	Ilu

Your patient has a methionine converted to arginine in his protein X. This happens to be in a transmembrane domain. Introducing a charged residue into a hydrophobic transmembrane domain is likely to cause major changes for the protein. Perhaps the altered protein is not able to be anchored in the membrane, for example.

c. Interaction of the T cells with the B cells is necessary for the B cells to progress beyond where they are making IgM. Without the assistance of the T cells, the B cells will not switch over from making IgM to making the other immunoglobulins. Hence there will be an immunodeficiency and an excess of IgM.

Your patient has X-LINKED IMMUNODEFICIENCY WITH HYPER-IgM.

References

Allen, R. C., Armitage, R. J., Conley, M. E., Rosenblatt, H., Jenkins, N. A., Copeland, N. G., Bedell, M. A., Edelhoff, S., Disteche, C. M., Simoneaux, D. K., Fanslow, W. C., Belmont, J., and Spriggs, M. K. CD40 ligand gene defects responsible for X-linked hyper-IgM syndrome. *Science* 259: 990, 1993.

DiSanto, J. P., Bonnefoy, J. Y., Gauchat, J. F., Fischer, A., and de Saint Basile, G. CD40 ligand mutations in X-linked immunodeficiency with hyper-IgM. *Nature* 361: 541, 1993.

Korthäuer, U., Graf, D., Mages, H. W., Brière, F., Padayachee, M., Malcolm, S., Ugazio, A. G., Notarangelo, L. D., Levinsky, R. J., and Kroczek, R. A. Defective expression of T-cell CD40 ligand causes X-linked immunodeficiency with hyper-IgM. *Nature* 361: 539, 1993.

CHAPTER 11

The Lungs

Problem 78

Your patient is a 40-year-old male nonsmoker with emphysema. You do a bronchoalveolar lavage and measure the elastase activity. You find that it is much higher than what you would expect for the lavage fluid of a normal person. You use chromatography to remove the elastase activity from the lavage fluid. You then add commercially available elastase to the lavage fluid and you measure elastase activity. The results are shown in Table P78-1.

a. In which protein is your patient defective? What does this protein do?

b. Why does your patient have emphysema?

TABLE P78-1

Source of Lavage Fluid	Elastase Activity (% of control)
Your patient	500
Normal person	100

Problem 79

Tobacco smoke contains oxidizing agents that oxidize certain methionine residues in α_1-antitrypsin. One of these is likely to be Met^{358}.

a. What is the protein with which α_1-antitrypsin normally binds?

b. How could these changes in the methionine residues lead to alveolar damage? What kind of disease will it cause?

Answer 78

a. After using chromatography to remove the native elastase from the bronchoalveolar lavage from your patient and from a normal person, you then add commercial elastase to the lavage fluid and measure the elastase activity in the fluid. You find that it is much higher in your patient's lavage fluid than in the normal fluid. This means that your patient must be defective in an inhibitor of elastase. The major inhibitor of elastase that would be present in the alveoli is α_1-*antitrypsin*. Hence this is likely to be the defective protein. α_1-Antitrypsin is an inhibitor of a wide variety of serine proteases, including trypsin, chymotrypsin, elastase, cathepsin G, collagenase, plasmin, and thrombin; elastase appears to be its favored substrate. Inhibition involves formation of a complex with the protease.

b. Elastase digests elastin, the major component of elastic fibers. These fibers play a major role in the lungs, causing the alveoli to shrink upon exhalation. If the elastic fibers are damaged, the alveoli will lose their elasticity and gas exchange will be compromised, leading to emphysema.

Reference

Cox, D. α_1-Antitrypsin deficiency. C. R. Scriver, A. L. Beaudet, W. S. Sly, and D. Valle (Eds.). *The Metabolic Basis of Inherited Disease.* New York: McGraw-Hill, 1989, Vol. II, Chap. 96, p. 2409.

Answer 79

a. α_1-Antitrypsin is an inhibitor of a variety of serine proteases, including chymotrypsin, cathepsin G, trypsin, plasmin, and thrombin. The protease most strongly inhibited by α_1-antitrypsin, however, is leukocyte *elastase*.

b. In normal α_1-antitrypsin, the side chain of Met^{358} projects into the substrate specificity pocket of elastase (Figure A79-1). The peptide bond which is set up to be cleavable is that between Met^{358} and Ser^{359}. What is not yet understood is why α_1-antitrypsin is an inhibitor but not a substrate. At any rate, the peptide bond is not cleaved and the protease

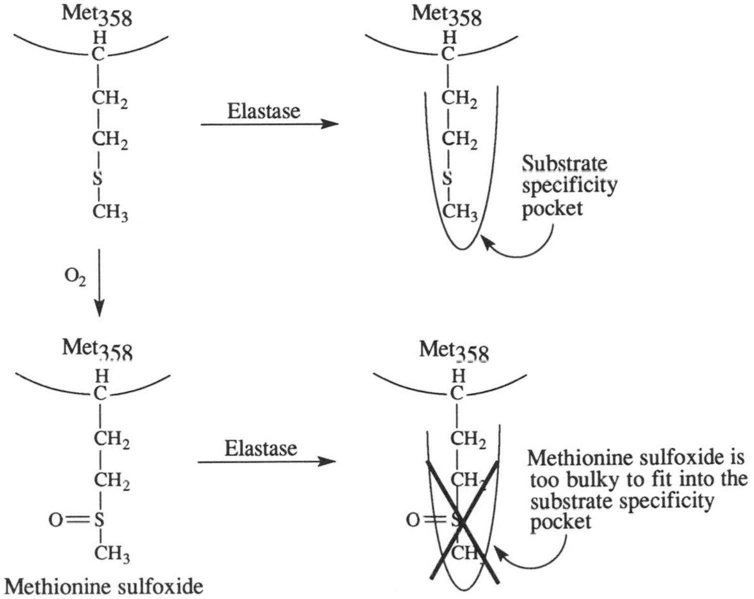

FIGURE A79-1. **Oxidation of Met[358] blocks the interaction of α_1-antitrypsin with elastase.**

remains bound to α_1-antitrypsin. When Met[358] is oxidized, the resulting methionine sulfoxide is too bulky to fit into the substrate specificity pocket of elastase. Its side chain is blocked by those of Thr[213], Val[216], and Thr[226]. The result is that the α_1-antitrypsin is no longer able to inhibit elastase. To be exact, its binding to elastase diminishes by a factor of about 2000. Thus the activity of elastase is significantly increased by tobacco. In addition, tobacco smoke is an irritant that increases the population of macrophages in the alveoli. These cells secrete a chemotactic factor that attracts leukocytes. Since leukocytes secrete elastase, the overall effect is to increase elastase activity greatly. Since elastase degrades elastin, the alveoli lose their elasticity, and the result is *emphysema*.

References

Beatty, K., Bieth, J., and Travis, J. Kinetics of association of serine proteinases with native and oxidized α-1-proteinase inhibitor an α-1-antichymotrypsin. *J. Biol. Chem.* 255: 3931, 1980.

Carrell, R. W., Jeppsson, J.-O., Laurell, C.-B., Brennan, S. O., Owen, M. C., Vaughan, L., and Boswell, D. R. Structure and variation of human α_1-antitrypsin. *Nature* 298: 329, 1982.

Cox, D. α_1-Antitrypsin deficiency. C. R. Scriver, A. L. Beaudet, W. S. Sly, and D. Valle (Eds.). *The Metabolic Basis of Inherited Disease.* New York: McGraw-Hill, 1989, Vol. II, Chap. 96, p. 2409.

Laskowski, M., and Kato, I. Protein inhibitors of proteinases. *Annu. Rev. Biochem.* 49: 593, 1980.

Loebermann, H., Tokuoka, R., Deisenhofer, J., and Huber, R. Human α_1-proteinase inhibitor: crystal structure analysis of two crystal modifications, molecular model and preliminary analysis of the implications for function. *J. Mol. Biol.* 177: 531, 1984.

CHAPTER 12

Connective Tissue

Problem 80

Your patient has very soft skin that is hyperextensible. She also has scoliosis. Biopsy of skin and cartilage reveals that the concentration of hydroxylysine in skin collagen is abnormally low, but that the concentration in cartilage collagen is normal.

a. Name the defective enzyme and describe what it does.

b. What kinds of collagen does the defective enzyme prefer as a substrate? (Be specific; use Roman numerals.)

c. Why does the defect produce abnormal collagen?

d. What is the vitamin cofactor required for the reaction catalyzed by the defective enzyme? Why is the factor required in our diet '(i.e., what enzyme do we lack that we cannot make this ourselves)?

Problem 81

Your patient has very soft skin, a hip dislocated since birth, and hyper-mobile joints. You culture her fibroblasts and find that they accumulate partly cleaved procollagen, namely collagen molecules still retaining the amino propeptide. You sequence the mRNAs for procollagen $\alpha2(I)$ and find that there are two mRNAs expressed in these cells. Their partial sequences are as follows (assume that the first nucleotide corresponds to the beginning of a codon):

1: GGCCCCCCUGGUCUCGGUGGGAACUUUGCUGCUCAGU
   AUGAUGGAAAAGGAGUUGGACUUGGCCCUGGACCAA
   UGGGCUUAAUGGGA
2: GGCCCCCCUGGUCUCGGUGGGGGGCUUAAUGGGA

mRNA 1 is the normal one. mRNA 2 has an abnormal deletion. (You have to figure out where it is.) You now obtain the procollagen $\alpha2(I)$ gene from your patient's fibroblasts and sequence it. You find that the sequence of *exons* of the coding strand of the gene corresponds *exactly* to the sequence of mRNA 1 (the normal mRNA). However, when you look at the sequence of one of the *introns*, you observe the following (exon is underlined):

Your patient: CAGTATGACGGAAAAGGAGTTGGACTTGGCCCTGGACCAATGGCATGCTTATCTG
Normal person: CAGTATGACGGAAAAGGAGTTGGACTTGGCCCTGGACCAATGGTATGCTTATCTG

You are able to sequence the N-terminal region of a tropocollagen $\alpha2(I)$ chain; the sequence is as follows, beginning with the N-terminal residue:

Gln-Tyr-Asp-Gly-Lys-Gly-Val-Gly-Leu-Gly-Pro-Gly-Pro-Met

Trace the etiology of your patient's problem from the abnormality in the intron to the poorly organized collagen fibers.

Problem 82

Your patient is a 28-year-old woman who bruises easily and who has hyperextensible joints. For example, she can bend her finger backwards until it touches the back of her hand. You find that her platelets do not aggregate in the presence of normal collagen, under conditions in which the platelets from a normal person would aggregate. You find that you can make her platelets aggregate in the presence of collagen if you add purified normal fibronectin.

    a. What is the defective protein in your patient?

    b. How does this defect explain the hyperextensible joints?

    c. How does this defect explain the easy bruising?

Problem 83

One of your patients recently died of an aortic aneurysm at age 33. You have cloned a portion of his DNA and identified the gene for fibrillin. You have sequenced the entire gene and compared it to the sequence of the fibrillin gene for a normal person. A portion of the gene sequences is as follows:

Codon number:	237	238	239	240	241
Normal person:	AGT	TAC	CGC	TGT	GAA
Your patient:	AGT	TAC	CCC	TGT	GAA

a. Speculate as to what the indicated mutation might do to the structure of the protein.

b. How might the alteration in fibrillin account for the aortic aneurysm?

c. Scientists are presently attempting to clone DNA from the hair of Abraham Lincoln; they are looking for a similar mutation. What characteristics of Abraham Lincoln could be explained by such a mutation?

Answer 80

a. Lysyl hydroxylase adds hydroxyl groups to certain lysyl residues in collagen. The reaction it catalyzes requires ascorbic acid and Fe^{2+} and is shown in Figure A80-1. The lysines that become hydroxylated are generally those on the amino sides of glycine residues. Type IV collagen is a particularly good substrate.

b. Lysyl hydroxylase favors as substrates collagens of types I, III, IV, and perhaps V.

c. Hydroxylysine forms more stable cross-links than does lysine. Also, the hydroxyl group is the site of glycosylation; the sugar residues may play a regulatory role in the cross-linking reactions, by which lysine and hydroxylysine residues are converted, respectively, to allysine and hydroxyallysine, which can then form cross-links among themselves and with histidine residues. These cross-links stabilize the collagen fiber.

d. The cofactor is ascorbic acid or vitamin C. The enzyme lysyl hydroxylase requires Fe^{2+}; ascorbic acid is necessary to keep the iron in the reduced state. Certain organisms, including ourselves, lack the enzyme L-*gulono-γ-lactone oxidase,* which catalyzes the last step in the pathway for synthesizing ascorbic acid (Figure A80-2); hence for these organisms, ascorbic acid is a vitamin. The pattern of which organisms have the enzyme and which lack it is rather complex. Among the have-nots are fish, insects, and many invertebrates. Amphibians, reptiles, and many,

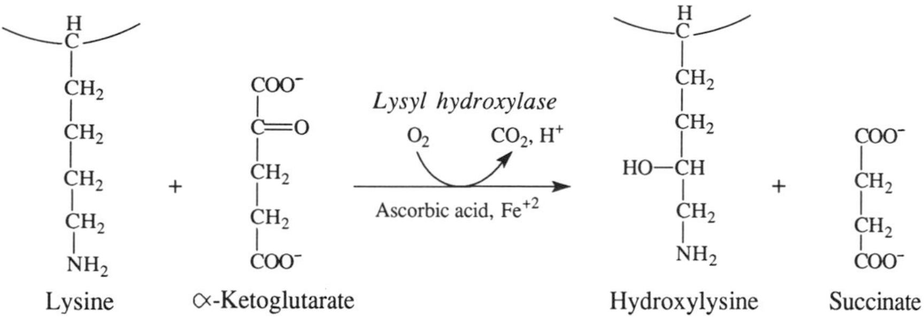

FIGURE A80-1. **Lysyl hydroxylase reaction.**

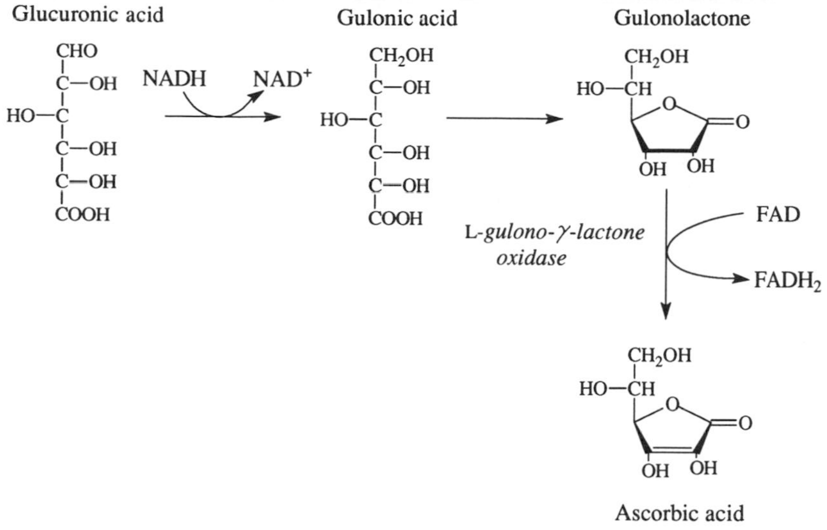

Glucuronic acid   Gulonic acid   Gulonolactone

L-gulono-γ-lactone
oxidase

FAD

FADH$_2$

Ascorbic acid

FIGURE A80-2. **Biosynthesis of ascorbic acid in nonprimate mammals.**

but not all, birds have the enzyme. Among the mammals, cows, goats, sheep, and rats have the enzyme, but not primates (including humans), bats, or guinea pigs.

Your patient has EHLERS–DANLOS SYNDROME, TYPE VI.

References

Bender, D. A. Nutritional Biochemistry of the Vitamins. Cambridge: Cambridge University Press, 1992, p. 363.

Byers, P. H. Disorders of collagen biosynthesis and structure. C. R. Scriver, A. L. Beaudet, W. S. Sly, and D. Valle (Eds.). The Metabolic Basis of Inherited Disease. New York: McGraw-Hill, 1989, Vol. II, Chap. 115, p. 2805.

Eyre, D. R., Paz, M. A., and Gallop, P. M. Cross-linking in collagen and elastin. Annu. Rev. Biochem. 53: 717, 1984.

Nobile, S., and Woodhill, J. M. Vitamin C. The Mysterious Redox-System: A Trigger of Life? Lancaster, UK: MTP Press, 1981, pp. 12–19.

Smith, E. L., Hill, R. L., Lehman, I. R., Lefkowitz, R. J., Handler, P., and White, A. Principles of Biochemistry: Mammalian Biochemistry. New York: McGraw-Hill, 1983, pp. 666–667

Answer 81

First try to find the deletion in the sequence of mRNA 2. To do this, scan along the two sequences until you see where they start to differ. Then detach the portion of the sequence in mRNA 2 beginning at that point and move it along until it lines up with the sequence of mRNA 1. This way you will see the deletion:

```
1:  GGCCCCCCUGGUCUCGGUGGGAACUUUGCUGCUCAGUA
    UGAUGGAAAAGGAGUUGGACUUGGCCCUGGACCAAUG
                                  GGCUUAAUGGGA
2:  GGCCCCCCUGGUCUCGGUGGG         GGCUUAAUGGGA
```

The deletion has the sequence

AACUUUGCUGCUCAGUAUGAUGGAAAAGGAGUUGGACUUGGCCCUGGACCAAUG

Now, determine the sequence of amino acids that the deleted region would have coded for:

mRNA: AAC UUU GCU GCU CAG UAU GAU GGA AAA GGA GUU GGA CUU GGC CCU GGA CCA AUG
Protein: Asn Phe Ala Ala Gln Tyr Asp Gly Lys Gly Val Gly Leu Gly Pro Gly Pro Met

Line up that procollagen sequence (A) with the N-terminal sequence of tropocollagen (B):

A: Asn Phe Ala Ala Gln Tyr Asp Gly Lys Gly Val Gly Leu Gly Pro Gly Pro Met
B: Gln-Tyr-Asp-Gly-Lys-Gly-Val-Gly-Leu-Gly-Pro-Gly-Pro-Met

In collagen biosynthesis, an N-terminal proteinase (procollagen amino-peptidase) cleaves procollagen to generate tropocollagen. Obviously, the cleavage takes place in the region of the sequence that you deduced was missing from your patient's procollagen, because the tropocollagen chain begins inside this sequence. If this region has been deleted, as is the case with your patient, the cleavage site has also been deleted. Hence your patient's procollagen will not be cleaved. Cleavage of procollagen produces tropocollagen, which then spontaneously polymerizes into collagen fibers. Without cleavage, collagen fiber formation will be inhibited and your patient will have soft skin, hyperextensible joints, and other joint problems.

Now you have explained the reason why the deletion causes problems. What causes the deletion in the first place? This is an intriguing question since the deleted portion of the procollagen is encoded in your patient's genome. Now, look at the sequence of the exons given above:

Your patient:	CAG TAT GAC GGA AAA GGA GTT GGA CTT GGC CCT GGA CCA ATG GCATGCTTATCTG
Normal person:	CAG TAT GAC GGA AAA GGA GTT GGA CTT GGC CCT GGA CCA ATG GTATGCTTATCTG
Exon mRNA:	CAG UAU GAC GGA AAA GGA GUUGGA CUUGGC CCU GGA CCA AUG
Protein:	Gln Tyr Asp Gly Lys Gly Val Gly Leu Gly Pro Gly Pro Met

Clearly, the exon codes for the deleted region. Thus the deletion described above occurred at the level of splicing and not in the DNA itself. The only difference between the DNA sequence of a normal person and that of your patient is that the normal person has a GT sequence in the intron immediately adjacent to the exon. In your patient that sequence has been altered to GC. It is known that for proper splicing to occur, there often needs to be a GT at the 5' end of the intron and an AG at the 3' end. In your patient's case, the GT is lacking and hence splicing is abnormal and the entire exon is deleted.

Your patient has EHLERS–DANLOS SYNDROME, TYPE VII.

References

Byers, P. H. Disorders of collagen biosynthesis and structure. C. R. Scriver, A. L. Beaudet, W. S. Sly, and D. Valle (Eds.). *The Metabolic Basis of Inherited Disease.* New York: McGraw-Hill, 1989, Vol. II, Chap. 115, p. 2805.

Weil, D., Bernard, M., Combates, N., Wirtz, M. K., Hollister, D. W., Steinmann, B., and Ramirez, F. Identification of a mutation that causes exon skipping during collagen pre-mRNA splicing in an Ehlers–Danlos syndrome variant. *J. Biol. Chem.* 263: 8561, 1988.

Wirtz, M. K., Glanville, R. W., Steinmann, B., Rao, V. H., and Hollister, D. W. Ehlers–Danlos syndrome type VIIB. Deletion of 18 amino acids comprising the N-telopeptide region of a pro-$\alpha2$(I) chain. *J. Biol. Chem.* 262: 16376, 1987.

Answer 82

a. Since the defect can be corrected by adding fibronectin, the defective protein is likely to be *fibronectin*.

b. Fibronectin is a major glycoprotein (440 kD) of the extracellular matrix. Fibronectin mediates collagen fiber adhesion to various cells. Defective fibronectin means less adhesive collagen, which means poorly organized collagen fibers and hyperextensible joints.

c. Platelets aggregate poorly and cannot bind well to collagen and to other cell surfaces; hence there will be less effective plugging of minor wounds, and that will lead to easy bruising.

Your patient has EHLERS–DANLOS SYNDROME, TYPE X.

References

Arneson, M. A., Hammerschmidt, D. E., Furcht, L. T., and King, R. A. A new form of Ehlers–Danlos syndrome. *JAMA* 244: 144, 1980.

Byers, P. H. Disorders of collagen biosynthesis and structure. C. R. Scriver, A. L. Beaudet, W. S. Sly, and D. Valle (Eds.). *The Metabolic Basis of Inherited Disease.* New York: McGraw-Hill, 1989, Vol. II, Chap. 115, p. 2805.

Answer 83

a. First, determine the results of this mutation:

Codon	237	238	239	240	241
Normal person:					
DNA:	AGT	TAC	CGC	TGT	GAA
RNA:	AGU	UAC	CGC	UGU	GAA
Protein:	Ser	Tyr	Arg	Cys	Glu
Your patient:					
DNA:	AGT	TAC	CCC	TGT	GAA
RNA:	AGU	UAC	CCC	UGU	GAA
Protein:	Ser	Tyr	Pro	Cys	Glu

Substitution of a proline for an arginine might disrupt an α-helix and alter the secondary structure of the protein in a major way. Also, the mutation takes place in a sequence of about 40 amino acids that is imperfectly repetitive, occurring 34 times in the entire sequence. The relevant portion of this sequence follows. (A sequence of five amino acids is shown; amino acids that are substituted in certain of the repeats are given underneath; the ones that occur most commonly are listed on top.

a	b	c	d	e
Gly	Ser	Tyr	Arg	Cys
	Gly	Phe	Lys	
	Thr		Glu	
	Leu		Gln	
	Lys		Thr	
	Asp		Ilu	
	Glu		Tyr	
	Asn		Asn	
			Met	
			His	
			Leu	

Although the precise role of this sequence in the function of fibrillin is not known, in none of the repeats is there a proline before the cysteine (at position d). This strengthens the argument that insertion of proline at this position is likely to be deleterious.

Fibrillin has some other strange properties. It has the rare modified amino acids hydroxyaspartate and hydroxyasparagine. It also binds several calcium ions, but the significance of this is not known. Interestingly, the mutation occurs in a domain that is thought to bind to calcium. If calcium plays an important role in fibrillin function, disruption of this domain by introduction of a proline may interfere with calcium binding and hence with the role of fibrillin.

b. Fibrillin forms microfibrils, along which elastic fibers are formed. An alteration in fibrillin could prevent normal elastic fiber formation. Since the aorta is the major tissue that contains elastic fibers, a weakening in these fibers could cause an aneurysm.

c. Fibrillin is a connective tissue protein. Although its roles are not all entirely understood, it is possible that an alteration in this protein could lead to the development of long limbs and long fingers, which Lincoln had. Fibrillin is found in the periosteum, a structure that normally constrains the growth of bones by maintaining some mechanical tension on the bone. When the periosteum is removed during surgery, bone growth is stimulated. It could be that a person with defective fibrillin will also have abnormally long bone growth.

Your patient has MARFAN SYNDROME.

References

Corson, G. M., Chalberg, S. C., Dietz, H. C., Charbonneau, N. L., and Sakai, L. Y. Fibrillin binds calcium and is coded by cDNAs that reveal a multidomain structure and alternatively spliced exons at the 5' end. *Genomics* 17: 476, 1993.

Dietz, H. C., Cutting, G. R., Pyeritz, R. E., Maslen, C. L., Sakai, L. Y., Corson, G. M., Puffenberger, E. G., Hamosh, A., Nanthakumar, E. J., Curristin, S. M., Stetten, G., Meyers, D. A., and Francomano, C. A. Marfan syndrome caused by a recurrent *de novo* missense mutation in the fibrillin gene. *Nature* 352: 337, 1991.

Dietz, H. C., McIntosh, I., Sakai, L. Y., Corson, G. M., Chalberg, S. C., Pyeritz, R. E., and Francomano, C. A. Four novel FBN1 mutations: significance for mutant transcript level and EGF-like domain calcium binding in the pathogenesis of Marfan syndrome. *Genomics* 17: 468, 1993.

Maslen, C. L., and Glanville, R. W. The molecular basis of Marfan syndrome. *DNA Cell Biol.* 12: 561, 1993.

McKusick, V. A. Abraham Lincoln and Marfan syndrome. *Nature* 352: 280, 1991.

CHAPTER 13

The Muscles

Problem 84

Your patient has Duchenne muscular dystrophy. He has had steady deterioration of muscle function since he was about 3 years old. Since the age of 13 he has been restricted to a wheelchair. He is mentally retarded. He will probably die from cardiorespiratory failure before he is 20.

a. Your patient has a defective protein, with a molecular weight of over 400 kD. What is the protein called? Describe the structure of the protein.

b. What is likely to be the function of this protein in a normal person?

c. Where is this protein located [organ(s), subcellular location]?

d. If the defective protein is critical for muscle function, why was your patient normal before he was 1 year old? *Hint:* Look at the paper of Tinsley et al. *Nature* 360: 591, 1992.

Note: The answer to question (b) is not yet known for sure. Nevertheless, some informed speculation would be appropriate here.

Problem 85

Two of your patients have Becker muscular dystrophy. Patient 1 is a 61-year-old man who has muscular weakness and needs a cane to walk. He is mentally normal and his cardiac muscle is unaffected. Using an antibody to the protein dystrophin, you find that your patient has normal amounts of dystrophin in his muscles but that the dystrophin is much smaller than normal. In fact, when you sequence his dystrophin gene, you find that it has a deletion that causes the protein to be 32% shorter. The deletion appears to extend from the first repeat segment to the thirteenth repeat segment.

Patient 2 is a 13-year-old boy who has some muscular weakness and easily gets cramps. When you look at his dystrophin and measure its molecular weight, you find that it is 600,000 D. Normal dystrophin is 427,000 D. The dystrophin gene of patient 2 has a duplication in the central repeat-rich domain of his dystrophin. The duplication is of the region encompassing the third to seventeenth repeat segments.

a. Speculate as to why your patients' diseases are relatively mild.

b. Speculate as to why they have any symptoms at all.

Problem 86

Your patient and her parents just moved here from Morocco. Your patient is a 2-year-old girl with severe muscular dystrophy. You do a muscle biopsy on the child and subject it to immunohistochemical analysis with an antibody to dystrophin. You find that dystrophin is present and appears to be normally distributed in the muscle; that is, it is associated with the sarcolemma. You purify the dystrophin; based on antibody binding and electrophoretic mobility, the dystrophin appears to be normal.

a. Assuming that the dystrophin is normal, what protein or proteins is/are likely to be missing from your patient?

b. What might be the role of the missing proteins?

Problem 87

Your patient underwent major surgery during which he was under general anesthesia. Shortly after the operation, he developed tachycardia; soon after that his temperature started increasing and his muscles became rigid. You are eventually able to bring his symptoms under control. Afterward you do a muscle biopsy; from the biopsied tissue, you prepare vesicles of the sarcoplasmic reticulum and load them with radioactive calcium. You then dilute the vesicles into a buffer and find that the rate of calcium release from the vesicles is much higher in your patient than it would be for a normal person.

a. How would the increased rate of calcium release from the sarcoplasmic reticulum cause muscle rigidity? Why would it cause the increase in body temperature? What might be the function of the protein that is altered in your patient?

b. How would you predict that ryanodine, a plant alkaloid that binds to calcium channels, would bind to your patient's vesicles compared to binding to those of a normal person?

c. A similar disease occurs in pigs, manifested by attacks when they are under stress. There is speculation that pig breeders, trying to create animals with lean meat, may have inadvertently selected for the defective gene. Explain this.

d. A veterinarian colleague has purified the sarcoplasmic reticula of both normal and diseased pigs. He finds that trypsin releases an 86-kD peptide from the sarcoplasmic reticula of normal pigs; the peptide is recognized by an antibody that is known to bind to the ryanodine receptor. This peptide is not released from sarcoplasmic reticula of diseased pigs. The N-terminal sequence of this peptide is Ser-Asn-Gln-Asp-Leu-Ilu-Glu-Asn-Leu.

When the genes from normal and diseased pigs were sequenced and compared, the following was found:

Codon number:	613	614	615	616	617	618	619	620
Normal pigs:	GCC	GTG	CGC	TCC	AAC	CAA	GAT	CTC
Diseased pigs:	GCC	GTG	TGC	TCC	AAC	CAA	GAT	CTC

Based on this information, how do you think the mutation could cause the defect in the protein? The answer to this is not known, so feel free to speculate.

Problem 88

Your patient is a 10-year-old girl who undergoes episodes of paralysis shortly after doing exercise. These episodes, which seldom last for more than 1 hour, are characterized by an inability to sit up or roll over without assistance. During these episodes, there is an elevation of serum potassium. The attacks can be precipitated by resting after exercise, by fasting, or by ingestion of potassium ion. You do a muscle biopsy and sequence the gene for her tetrodotoxin-sensitive sodium channel protein (Figure P88-1). You find that your patient has a mutation in this protein. The mutated sequence in your patient is shown below, together with the partial sequences from a variety of sodium channels in muscles of other organisms:

Your patient:	Tyr-Ilu- Ilu- Ilu-Ser-Phe-Leu-Ilu- Val-Val-Asn-Val- Tyr-Ilu-Ala- Ilu- Ilu-Leu
Normal person:	Tyr-Ilu- Ilu- Ilu-Ser-Phe-Leu-Ilu- Val-Val-Asn-Met-Tyr-Ilu-Ala- Ilu- Ilu-Leu
Rat:	Tyr-Ilu- Ilu- Ilu-Ser-Phe-Leu-Ilu- Val-Val-Asn-Met-Tyr-Ilu-Ala- Ilu- Ilu-Leu
Eel:	Tyr-Ilu- Ilu- Ilu-Ser-Phe-Leu-Val-Val-Val-Asn-Met-Tyr-Ilu-Ala- Val-Ilu-Leu
Fruit fly:	Tyr-Leu- Val-Ilu-Ser-Phe-Leu-Ilu- Val-Ilu- Asn-Met-Tyr-Ilu-Ala- Ilu- Ilu-Leu

Patch-clamp studies show that the sodium channel from your patient stays open considerably longer than that of a normal person.

a. What domain of the protein is the mutation likely to be in?

b. Why do you think that such an apparently minor mutation could have a large effect on the protein?

c. How could the mutant protein cause the paralysis?

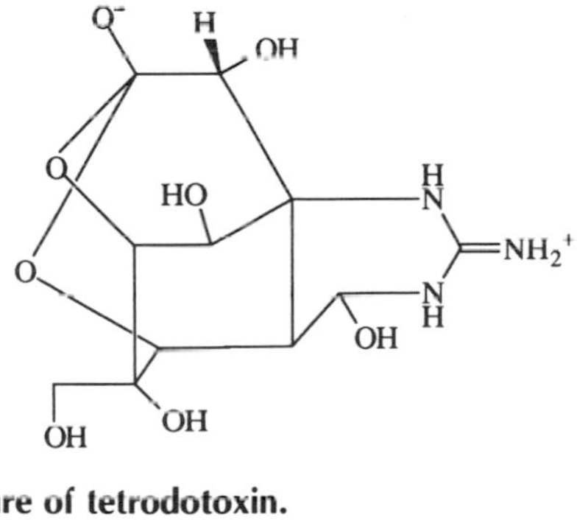

FIGURE P88-1. **Structure of tetrodotoxin.**

Problem 89

Your patient began acquiring fibrous deposits in his cornea when he was 25. When he was in his 40s the muscles on his upper face started to become paralyzed. He is now 72. The skin on his face and his back hangs in loose folds. He suffers from a great deal of itching. You biopsy some fibrous deposits from his kidney and sequence the peptide component. Here is the sequence of the N-terminal region of the peptide:

Ala-Thr-Glu-Val-Pro-Val-Ser-Trp-Glu-Ser-Phe-Asn-Asn-Gly

You use your repertoire of molecular biological techniques to sequence your patient's gelsolin gene. Here is a portion of the sequence, compared to that for a normal person. Codon divisions are shown.

Your patient: CGT GCC ACC GAG GTA CCT GTG TCC TGG GAG AGC TTC AAC AAT GGC AAC TGC TTC
Normal person: CGT GCC ACC GAG GTA CCT GTG TCC TGG GAG AGC TTC AAC AAT GGC GAC TGC TTC

A full sequence analysis shows evidence for a repeating domain structure of 125 to 150 residues. There are six domains. The first domain has been crystallized and its three-dimensional structure obtained. From this the structures of the other domains can be deduced. One could therefore predict that the structure shown in Figure P89-1 would occur in the interior of the second domain of gelsolin.

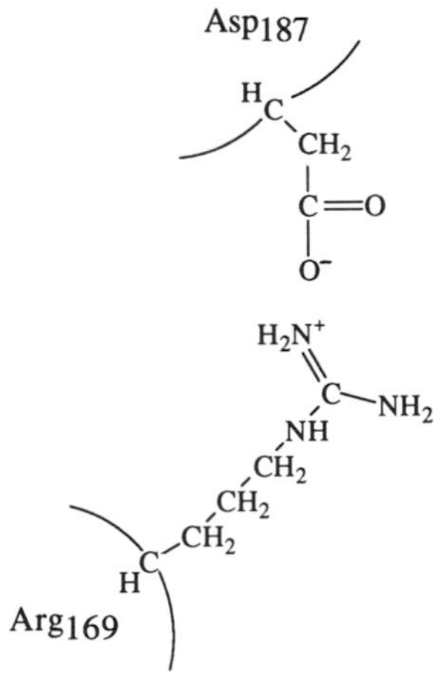

FIGURE P89-1. **Interior of gelsolin.**

a. Based on this information, how could the mutation in your patient lead to the fibrous deposits?

b. What is/are the functions of gelsolin?

c. Why does the disease not affect all of your patient's cells?

Answer 84

a. The missing protein is *dystrophin*. It has a molecular weight of about 427 kD and the open reading frame of its gene codes for a protein of 3685 amino acids. The N-terminal 200 or so amino acids have a sequence that resembles the actin binding domain of α-actinin, suggesting that this part of dystrophin may bind to actin. The C-terminal region of dystrophin appears to be involved in binding to some muscle membrane glycoproteins. Also, the C-terminal region contains what appear to be transmembrane helices, suggesting that the C-terminal region of dystrophin may be anchored in the sarcolemma. The central portion of dystrophin contains 24 to 26 repeating segments about 88 to 126 residues long and is predicted to form an α-helical coiled-coil structure. The dystrophin molecule is about 110 nm in length and 2 nm wide, with an overall dumbbell shape. It appears to form tetramers in a side-to-side staggered array.

b. The function of dystrophin is still not entirely clear. Here are some possibilities. It may be involved in organization of the thin filaments of the sarcomere or in anchoring of the thin filaments to the membrane or the transverse tubules. Dystrophin forms a complex with a membrane glycoprotein. This glycoprotein is bound to the extracellular matrix protein laminin, while the dystrophin binds to the intracellular actin. Thus dystrophin may participate in linking intracellular and extracellular skeletal proteins. Defective function of dystrophin thus disorganizes the cytoskeleton of muscle cells and its orientation or connection to the extracellular matrix. This leads to changes in the properties of the sarcolemma, which causes the muscle cells to die, leading to muscle atrophy. One possibility is that without the anchoring function of dystrophin, frequent stressing of a muscle cell may damage the sarcolemma.

c. Dystrophin is found largely in muscles: skeletal, cardiac, and smooth; of these skeletal muscle has about 10 times the level of the other two. Much lower levels, about 1 to 2% relative to that in muscle, have been found in brain, kidney, and lung. Even smaller amounts of dystrophin have been reported in liver, spleen, placenta, and fibroblasts. In muscle cells, it is localized on the cytoplasmic side of the sarcolemma.

d. There exists a dystrophin-related protein called *utrophin*. It is expressed in fetal muscle. It is similar in sequence to dystrophin, particularly in the C-terminal region, where the two proteins are 80% identical. This is the region to which the dystrophin-associated glycoproteins bind. The binding of these proteins appears to be an important function of dystrophin. Conceivably, utrophin is able to partially replace dystrophin in the neonate. Perhaps, as the child gets older, utrophin expression decreases and it is replaced by dystrophin. If the dystrophin is defective, problems arise.

References

Ervasti, J. M., and Campbell, K. P. A role of the dystrophin-glycoprotein complex as a transmembrane linker between laminin and actin. *J. Cell Biol.* 122: 809, 1993.

Love, D. R., and Davies, K. E. Duchenne muscular dystrophy: the gene and the protein. *Mol. Biol. Med.* 6: 7, 1989.

Sato, O., Nonomura, Y., Kimura, S., and Maruyama, K. Molecular shape of dystrophin. *J. Biochem.* 112: 631, 1992.

Tinsley, J. M., Blake, D. J., Roche, A., Fairbrother, U., Riss, J., Byth, B. C., Knight, A. E., Kendrick-Jones, J., Suthers, G. K., Love, D. R., Edwards, Y. H., and Davies, K. E. Primary structure of dystrophin-related protein. *Nature* 360: 591, 1992.

Answer 85

a. Dystrophin is a protein that appears to link together other proteins in the muscle cytoskeleton such as actin and certain membrane glycoproteins. If dystrophin is missing, there is very serious dysfunction of the muscles; this disease is called Duchenne muscular dystrophy. The regions of dystrophin to which actin and these glycoproteins bind appear to be the ends of the molecule. In each of these two cases, the dystrophin would still have the actin- and glycoprotein-binding sites to accomplish its basic functions.

b. Patient 1 is missing an interesting region located between the third and fourth repeat domains. This region (residues 668 to 717) contains five prolines in a row, making it impossible to constitute an α-helix. This is therefore a good candidate for a hinge region, allowing some flexibility and reorientation of actin filaments during muscle contraction. Patient 1 is missing this hinge region; his dystrophin may be less flexible than it ought to be. One can imagine that a less flexible dystrophin would either cause additional stress on the sarcolemma during contraction, which could lead to membrane stress on the sarcolemma during contraction, which could lead to membrane degradation and cell death, or else that it could cause misalignment of the actin filaments, thereby impeding contraction and causing weakness.

Although patient 2's dystrophin still has the key actin and glycoprotein binding site domains at the N- and C-terminal ends, he has greatly expanded the intermediate connecting region. Specifically, he has duplicated what is likely to be a hinge region (residues 668 to 717). If his dystrophin contains an extra hinge, it may be too "floppy" to orient the actin filaments properly with the extracellular matrix. This could therefore lead to excess stress on the membrane and some damage to the muscle cell.

References

Angelini, C., Beggs, A. H., Hoffman, E. P., Fanin, M., Kunkel, L. M. Enormous dystrophin in a patient with Becker muscular dystrophy. *Neurology* 40: 808, 1990.

England, S. B., Nicholson, L. V. B., Johnson, M. A., Forrest, S. M., Love, D. R., Zubrzycka-Gaarn, E. E., Bulman, D. E., Harris, J. B., and Davies, K. E. Very mild muscular dystrophy associated with the deletion of 46% of dystrophin. *Nature* 343: 180, 1990.

Koenig, M., and Kunkel, L. M. Detailed analysis of the repeat domain of dystrophin reveals four potential hinge segments that may confer flexibility. *J. Biol. Chem.* 265: 4560, 1990.

Love, D. R., and Davies, K. E. Duchenne muscular dystrophy: the gene and the protein. *Mol. Biol. Med.* 6: 7, 1989.

Answer 86

a. Some of the other forms of muscular dystrophy (Becker and Duchenne) involve deficiencies in the protein dystrophin. In this patient, the dystrophin seems to be normal. This is consistent with the fact that your patient is female, since defects in dystrophin are X-linked and appear primarily in males. Thus the defect is likely to be not in dystrophin but in a protein associated with dystrophin. These include the 156-kD dystrophin-associated glycoprotein, also called dystroglycan, the 59-kD dystrophin-associated protein, the 50-kD dystrophin-associated glycoprotein, the 43-kD dystrophin-associated glycoprotein, the 35-kD dystrophin-associated glycoprotein, and the 25-kD dystrophin-associated protein. In your patient, as in many others from North Africa, the 50-kD dystrophin-associated glycoprotein is missing.

b. These dystrophin-associated proteins form a transmembrane complex. The precise role of each protein in the complex is not clear. The 156-kD protein is thought to lie on the extracellular side of the complex and to be involved in binding to the extracellular matrix protein laminin. Loss of the 50-kD glycoprotein may disrupt the complex and prevent interaction between the actin filaments and the extracellular matrix, which may be the major function of this complex. Interestingly, when the 50-kD glycoprotein is missing, the other proteins are still present in the sarcolemma; this makes it likely that the 50-kD glycoprotein plays a major role in organizing the complex.

Your patient has SEVERE CHILDHOOD AUTOSOMAL RECESSIVE MUSCULAR DYSTROPHY.

References

Ben Hamida, M., Fardeau, M., and Attia, N. Severe childhood muscular dystrophy affecting both sexes and frequent in Tunisia. *Muscle Nerve* 6: 469, 1983.

Ben Jelloun-Dellagi, S., Chaffey, P., Hentati, F., Ben Hamida, C., Tome, F., Colin, H., Dellagi, K., Kaplan, J. C., Fardeau, M., and Ben Hamida, M. Presence of normal dystrophin in Tunisian severe childhood autosomal recessive muscular dystrophy. *Neurology* 40: 1903, 1990.

Ervasti, J. M., and Campbell, K. P. Membrane organization of the dystrophin–glycoprotein complex. *Cell* 66: 1121, 1991.

Matsumura, K., Tomé, F. M. S., Collin, H., Azibi, K., Chaouch, M., Kaplan, J.-C., Fardeau, M., and Campbell, K. P. Deficiency of the 50K dystrophin-associated glycoprotein in severe childhood autosomal recessive muscular dystrophy. *Nature* 359: 320, 1992.

Answer 87

a. Calcium plays a major role in muscle contraction. By binding to troponin C, it causes rearrangements in the tropomyosin and actin of the thin filament, thereby priming it to interact with the thick filament. Calcium can also bind to calmodulin and activate a myosin light chain kinase that will phosphorylate the myosin light chains (which are part of the thick filament) and stimulate their interaction with the thin filament. Finally, calcium binds to and activates phosphorylase kinase and the calcium/calmodulin complex activates a protein kinase that phosphorylates and inhibits glycogen synthase; the net effect of these last two is to increase glycogen breakdown greatly and thus increase the supply of energy available for contraction.

The increased concentration of calcium in the sarcomeres of your patient's muscles would cause the actin and myosin (thin and thick filaments) to interact at their maximal level, so the muscles would be maximally contracted and could not relax as long as the intracellular concentration of calcium remained high. The constant hydrolysis of ATP, without the performance of work, would cause the release of a substantial amount of heat and body temperature would increase.

It is speculated that the altered protein is involved in permitting calcium transport out of the sarcoplasmic reticulum into the sarcomere. This is consistent with your observation that your patient's sarcoplasmic reticulum vesicles are "leakier" to calcium. In your patient, the protein could be altered so that too much calcium is allowed to pass into the sarcomere.

b. Ryanodine would bind with higher affinity to these vesicles. Ryanodine (Figure A87-1) is an alkaloid from the plant *Ryania speciosa*; it has insecticidal properties. Ryanodine binds specifically to two gene products, both of which are calcium channels, one expressed in skeletal muscle and one in cardiac muscle and the brain.

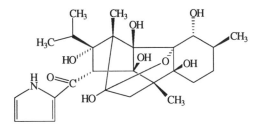

FIGURE A87-1. **Structure of ryanodine.**

c. Ordinarily, this is a gene defect that does not have deleterious effects. It is possible that in the case of the pigs, extra secretion of calcium into the sarcomeres may result in more contraction and oxidation of fuel reserves. This in turn would lead to leaner meat. Thus, in selecting for pigs with leaner meat, breeders may have been selecting for animals that had the defective calcium channel.

d. To understand how the mutation could have a deleterious effect, you must first look at the alteration in the amino acid sequence:

Codon number:	613	614	615	616	617	618	619	620
Normal pigs:								
DNA:	GCC	GTG	CGC	TCC	AAC	CAA	GAT	CTC
RNA:	GCC	GUG	CGC	UCC	AAC	CAA	GAU	CUC
Protein:	Ala	Val	Arg	Ser	Asn	Gln	Asp	Leu
Diseased pigs:								
DNA:	GCC	GTG	TGC	TCC	AAC	CAA	GAT	CTC
RNA:	GCC	GUG	UGC	UCC	AAC	CAA	GAU	CUC
Protein:	Ala	Val	Cys	Ser	Asn	Gln	Asp	Leu

The pigs with the disease have a cysteine replacing arginine at position 615 in the calcium channel protein. The sequence following the arginine is identical to the N-terminal sequence of the peptide released by trypsin from the sarcoplasmic reticula. Trypsin is known to cleave at lysines and arginines. Changing the arginine to a cysteine would prevent trypsin from cleaving here and from generating the 86-kD peptide. Hence the mutation must be in a region of the channel accessible to trypsin. Presumably, this would be on the external (cytosolic) side of the channel protein. Ryanodine binds to this peptide and hence to this region. It seems, in other words, that the mutation is in a region of the protein that is on the external (cytosolic) side of the channel protein. If the channel were subject to some kind of regulator, it is likely that the regulatory molecule would bind here. The mutation could therefore alter the ability to be regulated and cause the channel to be open all the time. This might not, however, explain the human disease, in which the mutation has not yet been identified. In your patient, the sarcoplasmic reticular vesicles are significantly more "leaky" to calcium, even when they are isolated and presumably separated from most other cellular components, probably including any hypothetical regulatory molecule. Another possibility is that the mutation either affects the structure of the channel itself, to make it "leakier," or increases the affinity of the channel protein for calcium.

Your patient has MALIGNANT HYPERTHERMIA. This is a potentially life-threatening condition for patients undergoing general anesthesia.

References

Budavari, S. *The Merck Index: An Encyclopedia of Chemicals, Drugs, and Biologicals,* 11th Ed. Rahway, NJ: Merck & Co., Inc., 1989, p. 1320.

Fujii, J., Otsu, K., Zorzato, F., De Leon, S., Khanna, V. J., Wiler, J. E., O'Brien, P. J., and MacLennan, D. H. Identification of a mutation in porcine ryanodine receptor associated with malignant hyperthermia. *Science* 253: 448, 1991.

MacLennan, D. H., and Phillips, M. S. Malignant hyperthermia. *Science* 256: 789, 1992.

Mickelson, J. R., Knudson, C. M., Kennedy, C. F. H., Yang, D.-I., Litterer, L. A., Rempel, W. E., Campbell, K. P., and Louis, C. F. Structural and functional correlates of a mutation in the malignant hyperthermia-susceptible pig ryanodine receptor. *FEBS Lett.* 301: 49, 1992.

Answer 88

a. This is a very hydrophobic region. Such a region is likely to be a transmembrane domain, since this is a membrane protein.

b. This entire region is highly conserved in evolution and the methionine that is mutated in your patient is completely conserved. Comparing the sequences of this protein with those from other organisms, you can see that several residues do not seem to mutate at all and the others undergo only very minor changes, such as Val ↔ Ilu or Ilu ↔ Leu. This underlines the conclusion that the Met → Val change in your patient could be deleterious. It is likely, therefore, that even a minor change at this position could disrupt the function of the protein.

c. The signal to begin skeletal muscle contraction requires a wave of depolarization to pass along the muscle surface. This involves rapid inactivation of sodium channels. If the sodium channels remain open too long, the system becomes leaky and the muscles will not register the signal to contract. There is clearly a connection to serum potassium here since attacks can be caused not only by potassium ingestion but by exercise and fasting, which also raise serum potassium. It is hypothesized that elevated serum potassium may cause a slight depolarization of the muscle cell which could lead, in a normal person, to entry of small amounts of sodium into the cell before the channel inactivates. In your patient, the lessened ability of the sodium channel to become inactivated would enhance the depolarization. It would also enhance loss of potassium from the cell, which would in turn raise serum potassium and create a positive feedback loop to make the problem worse.

Your patient has HYPERKALEMIC PERIODIC PARALYSIS (ADY-NAMIA EPISODICA HEREDITARIA).

References
Cannon, S. C., Brown, R. H., and Corey, D. P. A sodium channel defect in hyperkalemic periodic paralysis: potassium-induced failure of inactivation. *Neuron* 6: 619, 1991.

Gamstorp, I. Adynamia episodica hereditaria. *Acta Paediatr.* 45: 657, 1956.

Rojas, C. V., Wang, J., Schwartz, L. S., Hoffman, E. P., Powell, B. R., and Brown, R. H. A Met-to-Val mutation in the skeletal muscle Na^+ channel α-subunit in hyperkalaemic periodic paralysis. *Nature* 354: 387, 1991.

Stryer, L. *Biochemistry.* New York: W.H. Freeman and Company, 1988, p. 1013.

Answer 89

a. To understand the significance of the mutation in your patient, translate the nucleotide sequence into an amino acid sequence:

```
Your patient:
  DNA:     CGT GCC ACC GAG GTA CCT GTG TCC TGG GAG AGC TTC AAC AAT GGC AAC TGC TTC
  RNA:     CGU GCC ACC GAG GUA CCU GUG UCC UGG GAG AGC UUC AAC AAU GGC AAC UGC UUC
  Protein: Arg Ala Thr Glu Val Pro Val Ser Trp Glu Ser Phe Asn Asn Gly Asn Cys Phe
Normal person:
  DNA:     CGT GCC ACC GAG GTA CCT GTG TCC TGG GAG AGC TTC AAC AAT GGC GAC TGC TTC
  RNA:     CGU GCC ACC GAG GUA CCU GUG UCC UGG GAG AGC UUC AAC AAU GGC GAC UGC UUC
  Protein: Arg Ala Thr Glu Val Pro Val Ser Trp Glu Ser Phe Asn Asn Gly Asp Cys Phe
```

By looking up the sequence of gelsolin, you will identify this region as residues 172 to 189. Your patient has a mutation at position 187 in which an aspartate is changed to an asparagine (Figure A89-1). Why would such a seemingly minor change cause such a large outcome?

The x-ray structure of the first gelsolin domain shows that arginine 45 and aspartate 66 are oriented next to each other in the tertiary structure, and by deduction, arginine 169 and aspartate 187 should also be next to each other, in a position to form an ionic bond. Both arginine and aspartate are charged residues; the only way such residues could exist in the interior of a protein is if they are engaged in an ionic bond. The mutation of aspartate 187 to an asparagine, which is uncharged, leaves arginine 169 without a partner for an ionic bond. Hence arginine 169 has to move to the surface. This is bound to cause a change in conformation of the protein, which could by itself make it more susceptible to proteolytic degradation and aggregation. To understand this better, compare the sequence of the region of the gelsolin containing the mutation site with the N-terminal region of the protein which you have obtained from your patient's fibrils:

```
          172 173 174 175 176 177 178 179 180 181 182 183 184 185 186 187
Gelsolin:  Arg Ala Thr Glu Val Pro Val Ser Trp Glu Ser Phe Asn Asn Gly Asp
Peptide:       Ala-Thr-Glu-Val-Pro-Val-Ser-Trp-Glu-Ser-Phe-Asn-Asn-Gly-
```

Clearly, the peptide was formed by proteolytic cleavage at arginine 172. This cleavage site should not be surprising; there are plenty of proteolytic enzymes in the blood (coagulation and complement factors) which cleave polypeptide chains after arginine residues. Why does normal gelsolin not get cleaved at arginine 172? Probably because the arginine is oriented in some way so as to make it less accessible to proteolytic enzymes. However, in your patient, the movement of arginine 169 to the surface makes it very likely that the position of the nearby arginine 172 will be altered; the change obviously makes it more susceptible to proteolytic cleavage. Once the proteolytic cleavage has occurred, the resulting fragment aggregates to form the amyloid deposits. Precisely what feature of the structure of this peptide predisposes to aggregation is not clear.

b. Gelsolin exists in two forms: one is cytoplasmic and one is found in the plasma. The cytoplasmic form plays major roles in actin polymerization. Actin is the major protein of microfilaments, which consist of two strands of actin molecules wound around each other in helical array. In

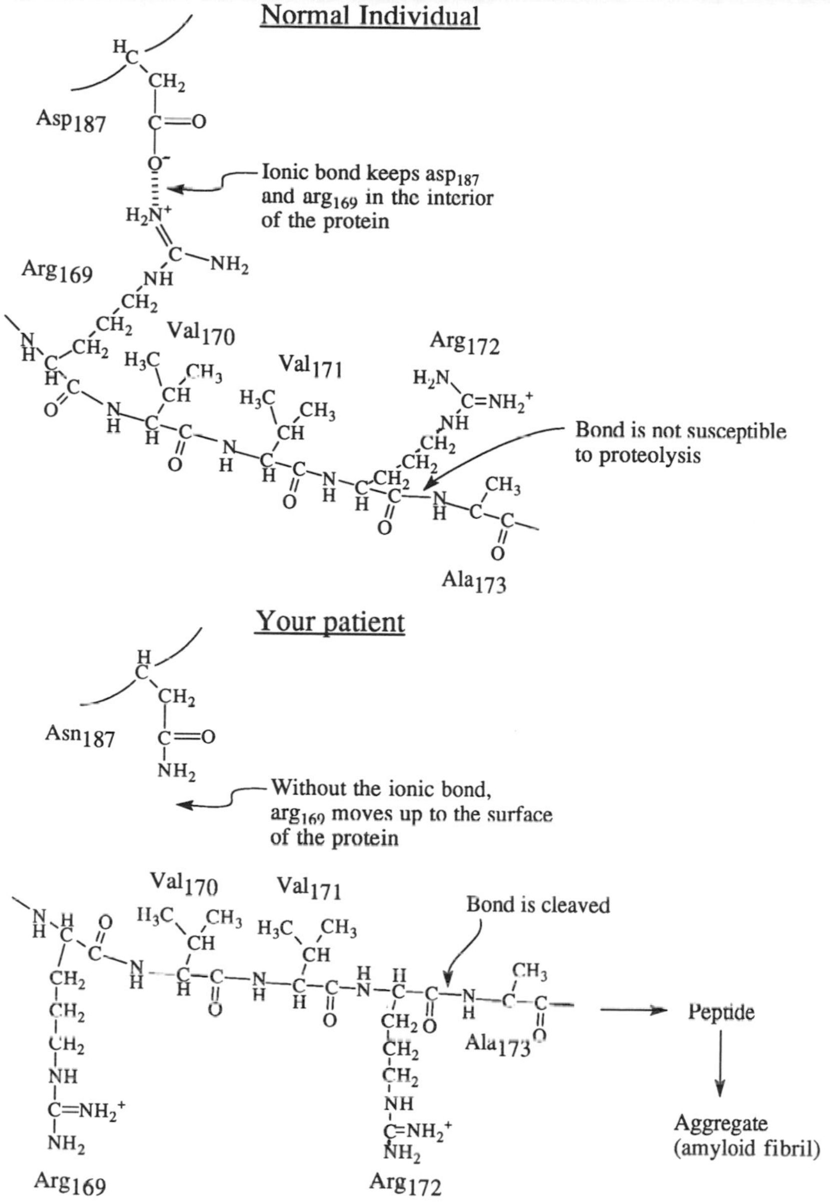

Normal Individual

Asp187

Ionic bond keeps asp187 and arg169 in the interior of the protein

H_2N^+

Arg169

Val170

Val171

Arg172

Bond is not susceptible to proteolysis

Ala173

Your patient

Asn187

Without the ionic bond, arg169 moves up to the surface of the protein

Val170   Val171

Bond is cleaved

Peptide

Ala173

Aggregate (amyloid fibril)

Arg169   Arg172

FIGURE A89-1. The $Asp^{187} \rightarrow Asn^{187}$ mutation makes gelsolin more susceptible to proteolysis.

many cells, the microfilaments form a subcortical array adjacent to the plasma membrane and act as a gel to give some rigidity to the cell shape. Gelsolin can sever actin filaments. The first domain can intercalate between consecutive actin molecules in a single strand of the actin double helix. This leads to disassembly of the actin filament and to the dissolution of the gel, hence the name *gelsolin*. This would permit cell movement, shape changes, and secretion of vesicles that have to pass through this area. Gelsolin's actin filament-severing activity is induced by calcium and inhibited by the phosphoinositides phosphatidyl 4-monophosphate and phosphatidylinositol 4,5-bisphosphate. Thus gelsolin plays a major regulatory role in cell movement, growth, and secretion. In addition, gelsolin, by virtue of binding to actin, can cap actin filaments and serve as a nucleation site for actin polymerization.

The plasma form of gelsolin is speculated to bind to and dissolve actin filaments that have been released into the plasma or the extracellular space as a result of tissue injury or cell death. This could be an important function since otherwise it is conceivable that these filaments could aggregate and precipitate.

c. If the explanation that you have derived above is true, why does all your patient's not gelsolin aggregate and cause trouble in all his cells? As mentioned above, there are two forms of gelsolin. They are identical except that the plasma form has an additional 25 amino acids. These two forms arise from two transcriptional initiation sites. A single cell can manufacture both sites. The mutation in your patient would therefore be in the cytoplasmic gelsolin as well as in the plasma gelsolin, which is the one that aggregates.

The reason why the mutation does not have even more serious consequences is twofold. First, the mutation does not appear to compromise the function of gelsolin seriously. It has been shown that to exhibit the actin-severing activity, it is necessary to have only the first domain of gelsolin plus 20 residues from the second domain, up through arginine 169, and not including aspartate 187. This would imply that aspartate 187 is not necessary for this activity, nor is it necessary to have the arginine 169 in the interior of the protein. Also, one calcium and one phosphoinositide-binding site are located in the first domain, suggesting that a mutation in the second domain might not affect the regulatory behavior of gelsolin. Nucleation of actin filaments involves the last three domains. The second domain (which includes your patient's mutation) and the third domain are involved in filament binding. Perhaps the mutation does not compromise this function. In short, the mutation may not interfere significantly with the functions of gelsolin.

The second factor moderating the disease is this. Even if the mutation in your patient's gelsolin makes it more susceptible to proteolytic digestion, the altered gelsolin may not encounter, in his cells, proteolytic enzymes that will cleave at arginine 172 and generate the aggregating peptide. Thus only the plasma form is likely to come into contact with the appropriate proteolytic enzymes.

Your patient has FAMILIAL AMYLOIDOSIS, FINNISH TYPE.

References

De la Chapelle, A., Tolvanen, R., Boysen, G., Santavy, J., Bleeker-Wagemakers, L., Maury, C. P., and Kere, J. Gelsolin-derived familial amyloidosis caused by asparagine or tyrosine substitution for aspartic acid at residue 187. *Nature Genet.* 2: 157, 1992.

Kwiatkowski, D. H., Mehl, R., and Yin, H. L. Genomic organization and biosynthesis of secreted and cytoplasmic forms of gelsolin. *J. Cell Biol.* 106: 375, 1988.

Kwiatkowski, D. J., Stossel, T. P., Orkin, S. H., Mole, J. E., Colten, H. R., and Yin, H. L. Plasma and cytoplasmic gelsolins are encoded by a single gene and contain a duplicated actin-binding domain. *Nature* 323: 455, 1986.

Maury, C. P. J., Alli, K., and Bauman, M. Finnish hereditary amyloidosis. Amino acid sequence homology between the amyloid fibril protein and human plasma gelsoline. *FEBS Lett.* 260: 85, 1990.

Mclaughlin, P. J., Gooch, J. T., Mannherz, H.-G., and Weeds, A. G. Structure of gelsolin segment 1-actin complex and the mechanism of filament severing. *Nature* 364: 685, 1993.

Meretoja, J. Familial systemic paramyloidosis with lattice dystrophy of the cornea, progressive cranial neuropathy, skin changes and various internal symptoms. A previously unrecognized heritable syndrome. *Ann. Clin. Res.* 1: 314, 1969.

CHAPTER 14

The Skin

Problem 90

Your patient suffers from a condition in which mild friction of his skin, predominantly but not entirely, on his hands and feet, can cause very painful blisters to arise. You do a skin biopsy; from the biopsy you isolate and sequence the gene for a protein called type I keratin K14. You observe the following mutation:

> Codon number: 384
> Normal person: CTG
> Your patient: CCG

a. Locate the mutation in the domain structure of keratin.

b. Speculate as to how this mutation could cause the observed symptoms.

c. You have a second patient with similar symptoms except that in his case, the blisters are restricted entirely to his hands and feet. When you carry out the same analysis as you did with the first patient, you find that the mutation is located in the gene for type II keratin K5. Your colleague says that these mutations should not matter, since a cell could form filaments out of either type of keratin. He says that the only person who should have symptoms is someone who has mutations in both type I keratin and type II keratin. What is wrong with your colleague's argument?

Problem 91

Your patient suffers from skin problems. In the area of his joints, hands, and feet, his skin resembles corrugated cardboard. As a child he had frequent blisters. You do a skin biopsy and treat the cells with an antibody to keratin. You find that in certain skin cells, the tonofilament network present in normal persons has disappeared and that the tonofilaments are in a disordered array around the nucleus. You analyze the gene sequences for his keratin proteins and find that the gene for type II keratin K1 is altered as follows:

Codon number:	308	309	310	311	312
Your patient:	GGA	GAA	CAA	AGC	AGG
Normal person:	GGA	GAA	GAA	AGC	AGG

When you measure the strength of interaction between your patient's type II keratin K1 and a normal type I keratin K10, you find that the interaction has increased by 10% over what you would find between normal keratin 1 and normal keratin 10.

a. What is the nature of the mutation in your patient; speculate on how the mutation might affect the interaction with keratin 10.

b. How might the mutation account for the blisters?

Answer 90

a. Keratin belongs to the family of the intermediate filament proteins. All of these have the same general structure: an N-terminal nonhelical domain, a large α-helical region, called the rod domain, and a C-terminal nonhelical region. There are several types of intermediate filaments (the number keeps growing). Types I and II are called keratin. The domain structure of type I keratins is as follows:

1. *N-terminal region.* This region is subdivided as follows. There is a fairly conserved segment about 15 to 30 residues long followed by a variable segment about 0 to 130 residues in length. In type I keratin K14, the N-terminal region consists of 115 residues total. It is very rich in serine (26 residues) and glycine (40 residues), including runs of up to six serines.

2. *Rod domain.* This region is also subdivided. First there is an α-helical 35-residue subdomain (called 1A), followed by an 11- to 14-residue nonhelical linker, called L1, followed by a second α-helical 93- to 101-residue subdomain (called 1B), then a 16- to 19-residue nonhelical linker (L12), then a short α-helical 19-residue subdomain (2A), then an 8- to 12-residue nonhelical linker (L2), and finally, a long α-helical 97- to 121-residue subdomain (2B).

3. *C-terminal region.* This consists of a highly variable region about 0 to 130 residues in length followed by a more conserved subdomain about 15 to 30 residues in length. In the case of type I keratin K14, the C-terminal region is 46 residues long. It resembles the N-terminal region in being rich in serine (11 residues), but it is not rich in glycine (2 residues).

The mutation in your patient is located in the middle of the α-helical domain 2B.

b. First, you need to identify the amino acid change arising from the mutation observed:

Codon number: 384
Normal person:
   DNA: CTG
   RNA: CUG
   Protein: Leu
Your patient:
   DNA: CCG
   RNA: CCG
   Protein: Pro

The α helices of keratin are involved in the formation of the keratin filament. Substitution of a leucine by a proline would cause disruption of this important α helix, meaning that the resulting filament would be very weak. The basal cells of the skin consist largely of these filaments. Mutations in keratin could disrupt the filaments. If the filaments are disrupted, the cells would be very weak and not resistant to even mild pressure. Their lysis could easily lead to blisters.

    c. Keratin filaments are obligate copolymers. In other words, they need to contain both type I and type II filaments. Mutations in either one could cause disruption of the filaments. The domain structure of type II keratins is very similar to that of the type I keratins, except that both the N- and the C-terminal regions contain additional conserved subdomains immediately adjacent to the rod domain.

Your first patient has EPIDERMOLYSIS BULLOSA SIMPLEX, KOEBNER FORM; your second patient has EPIDERMOLYSIS BULLOSA SIMPLEX, WEBER–COCKAYNE FORM.

References

Bonifas, J. M., Rothman, A. L., and Epstein, E. H. Epidermolysis bullosa simplex: evidence in two families for keratin gene abnormalities. *Science* 254: 1202, 1991.

Steinert, P. M., and Parry, D. A. D. Intermediate filaments: conformity and diversity of expression and structure. *Annu. Rev. Cell Biol.* 1: 41, 1985.

Wilson, A. K., Coulombe, P. A., and Fuchs, E. The roles of K5 and K14 head, tail, and R/K L L E G E domains in keratin filament assembly in vitro. *J. Cell Biol.* 119: 401, 1992.

Answer 91

a. The amino acid change caused by the mutation can be deduced as follows:

Codon number:	308	309	310	311	312
Your patient:					
DNA:	GGA	GAA	CAA	AGC	AGG
RNA:	GGA	GAA	CAA	AGC	AGG
Protein:	Gly	Glu	Gln	Ser	Arg
Normal person:					
DNA:	GGA	GAA	GAA	AGC	AGG
RNA:	GGA	GAA	GAA	AGC	AGG
Protein:	Gly	Glu	Glu	Ser	Arg

Keratin tonofilaments are heteropolymers between type I keratins (such as keratin K10) and type II keratins (such as keratin K1). The mutation (changing Glu to Gln) removes a negative charge. Could it weaken lateral interactions between keratin molecules in the tonofilament? Probably not, since the change appears to increase the ionic interaction between adjacent keratin molecules. The mutation thus appears to make the lateral interactions stronger. However, the mutation occurs just before the C-terminal end of the last α-helical subdomain in keratin (subdomain 2B). It is quite possible that this region may be involved in the head-to-tail (longitudinal) interaction between keratin molecules.

b. The mutation clearly does not interfere with heterodimer formation. However, it is located at the end of the keratin rod domain (positions 301 to 314). It could interfere with head-to-tail polymerization of the keratin molecules to make the filaments. Collapse of the filament networks could lead to cell death and blistering.

Your patient has EPIDERMOLYTIC HYPERKERATOSIS.

Reference

Rothnagel, J. A., Dominey, A. M., Dempsey, L. D., Longley, M. A., Greenhalgh, D. A., Gagne, T. A., Huber, M., Frenk, E., Hohl, D., and Roop, D. R. Mutations in the rod domains of keratins 1 and 10 in epidermolytic hyperkeratosis. *Science* 257: 1128, 1992.

CHAPTER 15

Eyes and Ears

Problem 92

Your patient is legally blind. She started out losing the ability to see at night, and gradually, over the course of 30 years, she became almost completely blind. Examination of her retina shows extensive degeneration of her rod and cone cells and deposits of retinal pigments around the midperipheral fundus. You have isolated and cloned your patient's peripherin gene. You find the following difference in the DNA sequences:

Codon number:	215	216	217
Your patient:	AAT	CTT	AGC
Normal person:	AAT	CCT	AGC

    a. What effect might this mutation have on the structure of the protein?

    b. How would an alteration in peripherin affect the retinal rod cell?

Problem 93

Your patient is deaf. He has a streak of white in his otherwise brown hair and he has white eyebrows. He also has a deformed bone structure in his face. From a sample of his DNA, using the appropriate probes, you have isolated and sequenced one of his homeobox genes (called HuP2). You find that there is a mutation which would affect position 21 in the predicted amino acid sequence. Shown in Table P93-1 is a portion of the sequence of your patient's homeobox gene product compared with that of a normal person and those of other homeobox proteins from other species.

a. How might this mutation affect the function of the protein? For clues look at the sequences in Burri et al. *EMBO J.* 8: 1183, 1989 (Figure 4) and Bopp et al. *EMBO J.* 8: 3447, 1989 (Figure 2); also look at Figure 3 in Hoth et al. *Am. J. Hum. Genet.* 52: 455, 1993.

b. How might an alteration in this protein bring about the symptoms of the disease?

TABLE P93-1

Source	Name of Protein	Amino Acid Residue Number							
		17	18	19	20	21	22	23	24
Your patient	HuP2	Ile	Asn	Gly	Arg	Leu	Leu	Pro	Asn
Normal individual	HuP2	Ile	Asn	Gly	Arg	Pro	Leu	Pro	Asn
Mouse	Pax 1	Val	Asn	Gly	Arg	Pro	Leu	Pro	Asn
Fruit fly	Paired	Ile	Asn	Gly	Arg	Pro	Leu	Pro	Asn
Fruit fly	Gooseberry	Ile	Asn	Gly	Arg	Pro	Leu	Pro	Asn

Answer 92

a. First identify the nature of the mutation:

Codon number:	215	216	217
Your patient			
DNA:	AAT	CTT	AGC
RNA:	AAU	CUU	AGC
Protein:	Asn	Leu	Ser
Normal person:			
DNA:	AAT	CCT	AGC
RNA:	AAU	CCU	AGC
Protein:	Asn	Pro	Ser

In your patient, a proline residue has mutated to a leucine. Although the three-dimensional structure of peripherin is not known, a mutation that changes proline to leucine is likely to play a major structural role. For one, since proline is a helix breaker, this change could allow an α-helix to extend or even to join with another α-helix. This could constitute a major disruption of the overall protein structure.

b. The function of peripherin is unknown. From its sequence, peripherin is deduced to be a membrane protein with four transmembrane domains, three cytosolic domains, and two domains in the lumen of the photoreceptor disk. The residue that is mutated in your patient is located in one of the intradisk domains. It is speculated that the cytosolic domains interact with cytoskeletal elements to provide some structure for the rod outer segment, without which the segment would collapse. The function of the intradisk domain is equally speculative. Treatment with tunicamycin (Figure A92-1), an inhibitor of protein glycosylation, causes a collapse of the rod disk. Both rhodopsin and peripherin are glycosylated, but only in their intradisk domains; this suggests that carbohydrate moieties may play a role in shaping the disks of the outer rod segments. The carbohydrate moioeties of rhodopsin and peripherin may interact with the carbohydrate moieties on the opposite membrane of the disk and cause adhesion. The glycosylated residue in peripherin is Asn[228], only 12 residues removed from the mutation in your patient. It is possible, therefore, that your patient's mutation may affect the orientation of Asn[228] in such a way that its function may be compromised. Also, the

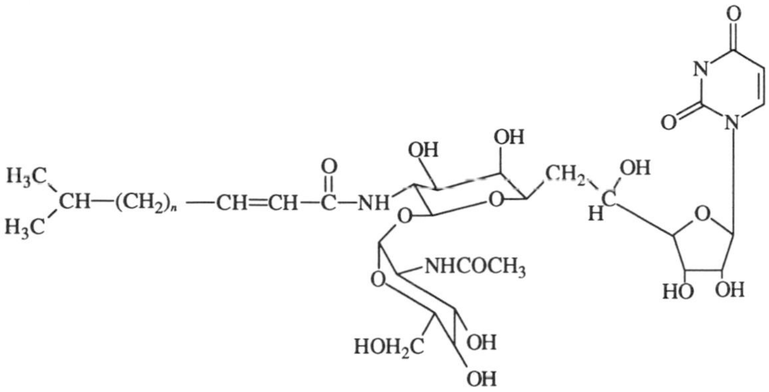

FIGURE A92-1. **Structure of tunicamycin. Tunicamycin is produced by**
Streptomyces lysosuperficus. **It is a mixture of related compounds, differing from
each other in their value of *n*. The major constituents are tunicamycins A, B, C,
and D, for which *n* = 8, 9, 10, and 11, respectively.**

intradisk domains of peripherin contain seven cysteine residues, some of
which are speculated to be involved in formation of disulfide bridges.
Three of these cysteines are located at positions 213, 214, and 222, very
close to the site of your patient's mutation. It is quite reasonable to
imagine that the mutation could alter the orientation of these cysteines
and disarrange or rearrange any disulfide bonds in which they may be
involved. This, in turn, could cause a large change in the structures of
the intradisk domains which could perhaps lead to collapse of the disc
and thus to blindness.

Your patient has RETINITIS PIGMENTOSA.

References

Budavari, S. *The Merck Index: An Encyclopedia of Chemicals, Drugs, and Biologicals,* 11th
Ed. Rahway, NJ: Merck & Co., Inc., 1989, p. 1544.

Bunker, C. H., Berson, E. L., Bromley, W. C., Hayes, R. P., and Roderick, T. H.
Prevalence of retinitis pigmentosa in Maine. *Am. J. Ophthalmol.* 97: 357, 1984.

Connell, G. J., and Molday, R. S. Molecular cloning, primary structure, and orientation
of the vertebrate photoreceptor cell protein peripherin in the rod outer segment disk
membrane. *Biochemistry* 29: 4691, 1990.

Kajiwara, K., Hahn, L. B., Mukai, S., Travis, G. H., Berson, E. L., and Dryja, T. P.
Mutations in the human retinal degeneration slow gene in autosomal dominant retinitis
pigmentosa. *Nature* 354: 480, 1991.

Answer 93

a. This mutation is very close to an α helix, spanning residues 27 to 35. Obviously, the proline at this position could not form part of an α-helix. Even mutating it to a leucine would not make it likely to participate in α-helix formation, because it is still between Gly[19] and Pro[23]. Therefore, it is not likely that the length of the α helix would be altered by the mutation. However, the proline at position 21 and much of the adjacent sequence is highly conserved in evolution, from which one can deduce that any changes would be deleterious.

Figure 3 in the paper by Hoth et al. is relevant at this point. Hoth et al. were working with PAX3, a homeobox protein related to HuP2. In PAX3, the sequence of residues 46 to 53 is Ile-Asn-Gly-Arg-Pro-Leu-Pro-Asn. This is identical to the corresponding sequence in HuP2. In PAX3, positions 53 and 54 are predicted to be part of a β turn (Figure A93-1). When position 50 (corresponding to position 21 in HuP2) changes from proline to leucine, the probability shifts and residues 49 and 50 are then more likely to form a β turn than are positions 53 and 54. This has the effect of changing the configuration of this region of the protein. Since the α helix is part of a DNA-binding helix-turn-helix motif, a change in configuration so close to the first α-helix may alter the DNA binding properties of the protein. Indeed, an analogous mutation in the same region in another homeobox protein greatly diminishes the ability of the homeobox protein to bind to DNA.

b. Homeobox proteins are DNA-binding proteins that appear to act as transcription factors. A mutation in this protein could have an effect in early embryonic life, altering the DNA-binding properties and affecting proper transcription of several genes and hence proper development of various characteristics. You would expect that a mutation in a transcription factor would have a variety of effects; that is indeed the case with your patient, who exhibits abnormalities in his hearing, facial bone structure, hair and eyebrows.

Your patient has WAARDENBURG'S SYNDROME.

References
Baldwin, C. T., Hoth, C. F., Amos, J. A., Da-Silva, E. O., and Milunsky, A. An exonic mutation in the HuP2 paired domain gene causes Waardenburg's syndrome. *Nature* 355: 637, 1992.

Normal

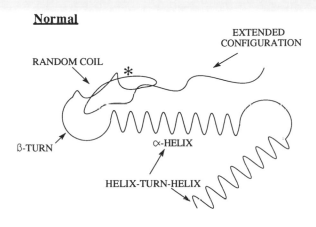

Mutant

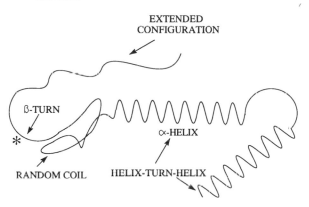

FIGURE A93-1. **Possible effect of a mutation on the structure of a homeobox protein. "*" is the site of the residue that is altered in the mutant.**

Bopp, D., Jamet, E., Baumgartner, S., Burri, M., and Noll, M. Isolation of two tissue-specific *Drosophila* paired box genes, *Pox meso* and *Pox neuro*. *EMBO J.* 8: 3447, 1989.

Burri, M., Tromvoukis, Y., Bopp, D., Frigerio, G., and Noll, M. Conservation of the paired domain in metazoans and its structure in three isolated human genes. *EMBO J.* 8: 1183, 1989.

Hoth, C. F., Milunsky, A., Lipsky, N., Sheffer, R., Clarren, S. K., and Baldwin, C. T. Mutations in the paired domain of the human PAX3 gene cause Klein–Waardenburg syndrome (WS-III) as well as Waardenburg syndrome type I (WS-1). *Am. J. Hum. Genet.* 52: 455, 1993.

Waardenburg, P. J. A new syndrome combining developmental anomalies of the eyelids, eyebrows and nose root with pigmentary defects of the iris and head hair and with congenital deafness. *Am. J. Hum. Genet.* 3: 195, 1951.

CHAPTER 16

The Gonads

Problem 94

Your patient is a 4-year-old boy who has the stature and physical strength of a boy of 8. His mental development is normal. When he was 2 years old, he began to develop pubic hair and his penis and testicles significantly enlarged. He suffers from a mild case of acne. Serum levels of testosterone are high, about what one would expect for a boy who has passed puberty. When you draw blood from his adrenal veins, testosterone levels are only slightly elevated. His father and grandfather exhibited similar symptoms, but none of his female relations showed any sign of precocious puberty. After going through various manipulations you isolate and sequence a gene that is altered in your patient. Here is the cDNA of a portion of your patient's gene, compared to that of a normal person's gene:

Codon number:	571	572	573	574	575	576	577	578	579	580	581	582	583	584	585
Your patient:	ATG	GCA	ATC	CTC	ATC	TTC	ACC	GGT	TTC	ACC	TGC	ATG	GCA	CCT	ATC
Normal person:	ATG	GCA	ATC	CTC	ATC	TTC	ACC	GAT	TTC	ACC	TGC	ATG	GCA	CCT	ATC

When you examine the entire sequence of the gene you find that there are discrete regions in the sequence which differ from each other greatly in the relative number of their hydrophobic residues (Table P94-1). You

TABLE P94-1

Region	Residue Number	Hydrophobic Residue
1	1–363	180
2	364–384	18
3	385–395	5
4	396–418	17
5	419–439	8
6	440–462	14
7	463–482	8
8	483–505	21
9	506–525	9
10	526–547	18
11	548–570	11
12	571–594	18
13	595–605	4
14	606–627	17
15	628–699	26

also notice that the sequences Asn-X-Thr and Asn-X-Ser in region 1 occur three times and two times, respectively.

Using the appropriate vector, you transfect this gene into a cultured cell line. You do the same with the normal gene. You measure the level of cAMP in each cell before and after addition of human chorionic gonadotropin (HCG) (1 μg/mL) to the culture medium. You also measure cAMP levels in a cell line which was transfected with the vector alone (without either the normal gene or your patient's gene). The results are listed in Table P94-2.

a. What is the altered gene in your patient?

b. How does the alteration lead to the symptoms?

c. Why do your patient's female relatives not exhibit precocious puberty?

TABLE P94-2

Transfection	HCG	cAMP (arbitrary units)
Vector alone	No	12
	Yes	12
Normal gene	No	12
	Yes	110
Your patient's gene	No	47
	Yes	110

Problem 95

Your patient is a 40-year-old man who has been married three times. Despite every effort, he never had children in any marriage. He is very susceptible to respiratory infections, particularly sinusitis and bronchitis. He is unusual in that he has his heart on the right side. He went to a fertility clinic and learned that the volume of his ejaculate is normal and the sperm number is also normal. His sperm are of normal appearance under the microscope and their metabolism is normal as well. The only unusual finding is that the sperm do not move. His sperm were embedded for electron microscopy and thin sections were generated and examined in the electron microscope. The results showed that the outer "arms," which in a normal sperm flagellum appear to go from one outer doublet microtubule to another, are missing in your patient.

a. What protein are the arms made of?

b. How does loss of this protein account for the immotile sperm?

c. What accounts for the high frequency of respiratory infections?

Problem 96

Your patient is a 20-year-old woman who has not menstruated. You gave her estrogen, which induced menstruation and caused her breasts to enlarge. Physical examination showed that external genitalia are female, pubic hair is sparse, and both clitoris and uterus are present. Further examination shows that the gonads are poorly developed. Karyotypy shows that she is XY and hence, genetically, male. Following biopsy, using the appropriate probes, you obtain the sequence of her/his SRY gene (located on the Y chromosome). Here is part of the resulting sequence, compared to that of a normal male:

Your patient: AAG   TAG   CTG
Normal male: AAG   CAG   CTG

a. How would this mutation affect the structure of the protein coded for by the SRY gene?

b. How could this bring about the resulting phenotype?

Answer 94

a. The altered gene is somewhere in the pathway that connects human chorionic gonadotropin to testosterone production. According to Table 94-2, in the transfected cells, the altered gene caused formation of cAMP even in the absence of human chorionic gonadotropin. Hence we have a system that is partly turned on even in the absence of a hormone. The alteration must be in either the receptor, G protein, or adenyl cyclase. Adenyl cyclase is the least likely candidate, because if adenyl cyclase was altered so as to be either more active or to be expressed more, one would expect that cAMP levels would be higher than normal even after hormonal stimulation. Instead, you see high levels in the absence and normal levels in the presence of hormone.

A close look at the cDNA comparison helps us to identify the altered protein. Convert Table P94-1 as shown in Table A94-1. It is clear from this analysis that the gene in question has a series of discrete hydrophobic segments (regions 2, 4, 6, 8, 10, 12, and 14) 21 to 24 residues long. These have the appearance of transmembrane segments. Also, the Asn-X-Ser and Asn-X-Thr segments in region 1 suggests that these could be attachment points for oligosaccharides. Since oligosaccharides are generally attached to extracellular domains, region 1 is likely to be extra-cellular. A protein that has an extracellular domain followed by a series

TABLE A94-1

Region	Length of Segment	Percent Hydrophobic Residue
1	363	50
2	21	86
3	11	45
4	23	74
5	21	38
6	23	61
7	20	40
8	23	91
9	20	45
10	22	82
11	23	48
12	24	75
13	11	36
14	22	77
15	72	36

of transmembrane segments must be a receptor. Hence the altered protein in your patient is a receptor.

What is it a receptor for? The experiment whose results are given in Table P94-2 would suggest that this is a receptor for human chorionic gonadotropin. It turns out, however, that the same protein is also a receptor for luteinizing hormone. In males, this is a more important hormone than human chorionic gonadotropin. Hence we can conclude that the altered protein is *luteinizing hormone receptor*. This would also explain why the adrenals are not making excess testosterone, which, if they were, would indicate some alteration in steroid metabolism in the adrenals. Everything points to a defect in the Leydig cells of the testis, which are the ones that make testosterone in response to luteinizing hormone.

b. To see how the alteration could lead to the symptoms, we first have to identify the nature of the mutation. This can be done as follows:

Codon number:	571	572	573	574	575	576	577	578	579	580	581	582	583	584	585
Your patient:															
cDNA:	ATG	GCA	ATC	CTC	ATC	TTC	ACC	GGT	TTC	ACC	TGC	ATG	GCA	CCT	ATC
mRNA:	AUG	GCA	AUC	CUC	AUC	UUC	ACC	GGU	UUC	ACC	UGC	AUG	GCA	CCU	AUC
Protein:	Met	Ala	Ilu	Leu	Ilu	Phe	Thr	Gly	Phe	Thr	Cys	Met	Ala	Pro	Ilu
Normal person:															
cDNA:	ATG	GCA	ATC	CTC	ATC	TTC	ACC	GAT	TTC	ACC	TGC	ATG	GCA	CCT	ATC
mRNA:	AUG	GCA	AUC	CUC	AUC	UUC	ACC	GAU	UUC	ACC	UGC	AUG	GCA	CCU	AUC
Protein:	Met	Ala	Ilu	Leu	Ilu	Phe	Thr	Asp	Phe	Thr	Cys	Met	Ala	Pro	Ilu

The mutation in your patient's receptor gene is the replacement of an adenine by a guanine, leading to replacement of an aspartate by a glycine at position 578 in a transmembrane segment. When a hormone binds to its receptor, it induces a conformational change in the extracellular domain which is transmitted through the transmembrane segments and then to the intracellular domains, leading to the activation of a G protein, which in turn activates adenyl cyclase. It appears that replacing the aspartate by a glycine leads to a conformational change which results in partial activity. Hence the presence of glycine must somehow be conducive to the conformational change. What is the difference between glycine and aspartate? Aspartate is capable of forming both electrostatic and hydrogen bonds, whereas glycine is not; glycine is also very small. The fact that aspartate 578 is one of the few hydrophilic amino acids in a hydrophobic domain underlines its importance. Perhaps the conformational change induced by the hormone involves breaking these electrostatic or hydrogen bonds. In the presence of glycine, the bonds would not be there and the conformational change would be partly complete at all times. Also, a segment of a polypeptide containing glycine instead of aspartate may be more mobile because the absence of a side chain in the glycine decreases steric hindrance and makes it easier for the conformation of the chain to change.

This receptor plays a crucial role in the changes that characterize puberty. When the levels of luteinizing hormone increase in males, it binds to this receptor in Leydig cells and causes them to secrete more testosterone. The testosterone, in turn, targets certain cells and causes the changes in secondary sexual characteristics that are associated with puberty. In your patient, the receptor is in its active conformation even in the absence of luteinizing hormone; hence the child exhibits signs of puberty even as a toddler.

c. The syndrome that your patient has is clearly inherited. The reason the females in his family do not have the syndrome is that the changes associated with puberty in women require both luteinizing hormone and follicle-stimulating hormone. Thus even if a woman has an altered receptor for luteinizing hormone which is always in an active conformation, few changes would be noted as long as follicle-stimulating hormone is at prepubertal levels.

Your patient has FAMILIAL MALE PRECOCIOUS PUBERTY.

References

Jia, X.-C., Oikawa, M., Bo, M., Tanaka, T., Ny, T., Boime, I., and Hsueh, A. J. W. Expression of human luteinizing hormone (LH) receptor: interaction with LH and chorionic gonadotropin from human but not equine, rat, and ovine species. *Mol. Endocrinol.* 5: 759, 1991.

Minegishi, T., Nakamura, K., Takakura, Y., Miyamoto, K., Hasegawa, Y., Ibuki, Y., and Igarashi, M. Cloning and sequencing of human LH/hCG receptor cDNA. *Biochem. Biophys. Res. Commun.* 172: 1049, 1990.

Rosenthal, S. M., Grumbach, M. M., and Kaplan, S. L. Gonadotropin-independent familial sexual precocity with premature Leydig and germinal cell maturation (familial testotoxicosis): effects of a potent luteinizing hormone-releasing factor agonist and medroxyprogesterone acetate therapy in four cases. *J. Clin. Endocrinol. Metab.* 57: 571, 1983.

Shenker, A., Laue, L., Kosugi, S., Merendino, J. J., Minegishi, T., and Cutler, G. B. A constitutively activating mutation of the luteinizing hormone receptor in familial male precocious puberty. *Nature* 365: 652, 1993.

Walker, S. H. Constitutional true sexual precocity. *J. Pediatr.* 41: 251, 1952.

Answer 95

a. The outer doublet microtubules of the axonemes of functional cilia and many flagella have both inner arms and outer arms at intervals along their length, the outer arms occurring every 24 nm and the inner arms in groups of three which repeat every 96 nm. The dynein arms are bound to the A-tubule of the outer doublet. The arms are made of *axonemal dynein.* Dynein is a large protein (MW 1,250,000). It has not been well characterized in humans or even in mammals. Of the well-characterized outer arm dyneins, the most closely related to humans is that from the trout, which is composed of two large polypeptides (415 and 430 kD), five intermediate-size polypeptides (57, 63, 65, 73, and 85 kD), and six small polypeptides (6, 7.5, 9, 11.5, 19, and 22 kD). There are about seven to nine different isoforms of the large polypeptide. The dyneins of the inner arms are distinct from the dyneins of the outer arms. In addition, many tissues contain a different protein, cytoplasmic dynein.

Presumably, in your patient, either there is a defect in one of these subunits and therefore the dynein complex is unable to bind to the outer doublet or else there is a defect in a protein that may help to organize the axoneme.

b. All dyneins are ATPases. They hydrolyze bound ATP and use the energy for motility. In a sense the dynein arm that is bound to the A-tubule of the outer doublet uses this energy to "walk" on the B-tubule of the adjacent outer doublet. This causes the outer doublets to slide with respect to one another. In an intact cilium or flagellum the movement is highly organized, so that at any given instant, the sliding is done largely by outer doublets on one side of the axoneme. This has the effect of causing the bending of the flagellum or cilium, which is the basis of their waving or whiplike motion. If the dynein arms are missing, the axoneme cannot bend and the flagellum is immotile and the sperm cannot move.

c. Presumably the defective polypeptide is part of, or associated with, all the axonemal dyneins in your patient. The cilia of the respiratory tract also contain axonemes with dynein arms. In your patient, these cilia would be immotile and hence be unable to expel foreign particles. This would naturally lead to a high frequency of respiratory infections. An intriguing question is why his internal organs are reversed (*situs* *inversus lateralis*). Many patients with your patient's disease also have their internal organs reversed. Perhaps very early in embryonic develop- ment, there may be a stage where cilia, powered by dynein, act to organize the positions of the future organs. If the cilia are immotile, the organization may become more random.

Your patient has KARTAGENER'S SYNDROME.

References

Afzelius, B. A. A human syndrome caused by immotile cilia. *Science* 193: 317, 1976.

Afzelius, B. A., and Mossberg, B. Immotile cilia syndrome (primary ciliary dyskenesia), including Kartagener syndrome. C. R. Scriver, A. L. Beaudet, W. S. Sly, and D. Valle (Eds.). *The Metabolic Basis of Inherited Disease.* New York: McGraw-Hill, 1989, Vol. II, Chap. 112, p. 2739.

Holzbaur, E. L. F., Mikami, A., Paschal, B. M., and Vallee, R. B. Molecular characteriza- tion of cytoplasmic dynein. J. S. Hyams and C. W. Lloyd (Eds.). *Microtubules.* New York: Wiley-Liss, 1994, p. 251.

Smith, E. F., and Sale, W. S. Structural and functional reconstitution of inner dynein arms in *Chlamydomonas* flagellar axonemes. *J. Cell Biol.* 117: 573, 1992.

Witman, G. B., Wilkerson, C. G., and King, S. M. The biochemistry, genetics, and molecular biology of flagellar dynein. J. S. Hyams and C. W. Lloyd (Eds.). *Microtu- bules.* New York: Wiley-Liss, 1994, p. 229.

Answer 96

a. First, turn the DNA sequence into a protein sequence:

Your patient:

DNA:	AAG	TAG	CTG
RNA:	AAG	UAG	CUG
Protein:	Lys	STOP	***

Normal male:

DNA:	AAG	CAG	CTG
RNA:	AAG	CAG	CUG
Protein:	Lys	Gln	Leu

Your patient has a nonsense mutation, introducing a STOP codon into the mRNA. This would cause the SRY protein to be made only in truncated form and hence to be inactive.

b. SRY stands for "sex-determining region Y." The SRY gene product is hypothesized to bind to DNA and inhibit the synthesis of an as yet undiscovered protein called "Z." Z protein inhibits the synthesis of the male-specific genes, such as the ones creating the testis. In a normal male, the synthesis of the SRY protein would prevent the synthesis of Z protein; without Z protein, the male-specific genes would be expressed. In a normal female, the SRY gene is missing; thus the Z protein is made and inhibits expression of the male-specific genes. In your patient the truncated SRY gene product would be unable to bind to DNA, and hence Z protein would be synthesized and would repress expression of the male-specific genes. Thus no testis would form and the affected person would appear to be female. There are also XX individuals who appear to be male. It is hypothesized that these individuals, who obviously lack the SRY gene, have a defect in the Z protein gene so that the Z protein is either inactive or not expressed. Without the Z protein, these people would appear to be male.

References

Harley, V. R., Jackson, D. I., Hextall, P. J., Hawkins, J. R., Berkovitz, G. D., Sockanathan, S., Lovell-Badge, R., and Goodfellow, P. N. DNA binding activity of recombinant SRY from normal males and XY females. *Science* 255: 453, 1992.

McElreavey, K., Vilain, E., Abbas, N., Herskowitz, I., and Fellous, M. A regulatory cascade hypothesis for mammalian sex determination: SRY represses a negative regulator of male development. *Proc. Natl. Acad. Sci. USA* 90: 3368, 1993.

McElreavey, K., Vilain, E., Boucekkine, C., Vidaud, M., Jaubert, F., Richaud, F., and Fellous, M. XY sex reversal associated with a nonsense mutation in SRY. *Genomics* 13: 838, 1992.

Sinclair, A. H., Berta, P., Palmer, M. S., Hawkins, J. R., Griffiths, B. L., Smith, M. J., Foster, J. W., Frischauf, A.-M., Lovell-Badge, R., and Goodfellow, P. N. A gene from the human sex-determining region encodes a protein with homology to a conserved DNA-binding motif. *Nature* 346: 240, 1990.

CHAPTER 17

The Brain and Nervous System

Problem 97

Your patient was a 36-year-old woman who just died of a massive brain hemorrhage. The autopsy of the brain shows large amounts of a fibrous deposit in her cerebral arteries. Your analysis of these deposits indicates that they are made of cystatin C. You sequence the cystatin C and find that its N-terminal sequence differs from that of a normal person as follows:

Your patient: Gly Gly Pro Met Asp Ala Ser Val
Normal person: Ser Ser Pro Gly Lys Pro Pro Arg Leu Val Gly Gly Pro Met Asp Ala Ser Val

You collect some of your patient's RNA using the appropriate probe; you then make the cDNA and sequence it. Here is the sequence of your patient's cDNA for cystatin C:

Codon number:	−26	−25	−24	−23	1	2	3	4	66	67	68	69	70
Your patient:	ATG	GCC	GGG	CCC. . .	TCC	AGT	CCC	GGC. . .	GTG	GAG	CAG	GGC	CGA
Normal person:	ATG	GCC	GGG	CCC. . .	TCC	AGT	CCC	GGC. . .	GTG	GAG	CTG	GGC	CGA

Unfortunately, you were not able to help the patient, but you find that you could use the restriction endonuclease *Alu*I to test your patient's children for the likelihood of developing the disease later.

a. What is the normal role of cystatin C?

b. Speculate on how the mutation at position 68 could lead to deposition of truncated cystatin C.

c. Why is *Alu*I useful in developing a test for the presence of the mutation?

Problem 98

Your patient is a 40-year-old Dutch man who has just died of cerebral hemorrhage, the last of several. He has had several relatives who have also died of this disease. Autopsy reveals the presence of a fibrous deposit in the blood vessels of his cerebral cortex. The fibrous deposit contains a peptide of 39 amino acids which you sequence, obtaining the following results:

Residue number:	16	17	18	19	20	21	22	23	24	25	26	27	28
Peptide:	Lys	Leu	Val	Phe	Phe	Ala	Gln	Asp	Val	Gly	Ser	Asn	Lys

The 39-amino acid peptide, which contains 22 hydrophobic amino acids and 9 charged amino acids, is not found in normal persons.

You obtain the sequence of the gene coding for a much larger protein called β-amyloid precursor protein (BAPP), which is involved in Alzheimer's disease:

Codon number:	1	2	3	4	5	. . .	612	613	614	615	616	617	618	619	620	621	622	623	624
BAPP:	ATG	CTG	CCC	GGT	TTG	. . .	AAA	TTG	GTG	TTC	TTT	GCA	GAA	GAT	GTG	GGT	TCA	AAC	AAA

Based on your analyses, you decide that the restriction endonuclease MboII could be used to screen members of your patient's family to see if they are likely to develop the same disease.

a. Is there a mutation, and if so, how might the mutation account for the disease?

b. Why would MboII be a useful screening tool?

Problem 99

Your patient has just died at the age of 76 after several years of progressive memory loss and dementia. Upon autopsy, you discover that she has cerebral deposits of a small protein about 40 amino acids long. You sequence this protein and find that it has the N-terminal sequence Asp-Ala-Glu-Phe-Arg. You isolate and sequence a gene for a certain large protein in both your patient and in a normal person. Here is a partial sequence:

Codon number:	589	590	591	592	593	594	595	596	597	598	599	600	601
Your patient:	GAG	GAG	ATC	TCT	GAA	GTG	AAT	CTG	GAT	GCA	GAA	TTC	CGA
Normal person:	GAG	GAG	ATC	TCT	GAA	GTG	AAG	ATG	GAT	GCA	GAA	TTC	CGA

a. What are these proteins?

b. How might the mutation in the protein sequence shown above cause the deposition of the small protein, and how might this cause the symptoms of the disease?

Problem 100

Your patient was a boy born with a small head, pinched cheeks, and receding jaw. He was cyanotic at birth and experienced several episodes of cyanosis during his 4 months of life. He exhibited failure to thrive and was very lethargic. He had difficulty swallowing and often aspirated his breast milk. After he died at the age of 4 months, an autopsy showed that the surface of his brain was much smoother than normal, lacking many convolutions, and that his brain weighed 70% of normal. You look at certain cDNA clones corresponding to genes from chromosome 17. You find that your patient had a deletion in a gene. You are able to obtain the sequence of the gene from a normal person, although the function of the gene is not known. By studying the sequence of the gene for which the protein codes and comparing it to those of certain other proteins, you make the following observations.

First, the sequence of the protein has a series of eight imperfect repeats, each one about 40 amino acids long, except for number 8, which is truncated and only 16 amino acids long. The structure of the protein can be diagrammed as follows:

$$N — R_1 — R_2 — R_3 — R_4 — R_5 — X — R_6 — R_7 — R_8,$$

where N stands for an N-terminal region, not repeated; R_1, R_2, and so on, stand for the different repeats; and X stands for an unrepeated segment of 20 amino acids inserted between repeats 5 and 6.

As you search the databases for similar proteins, you find three that are possibly related.

1. Human β-*transducin* has 55% sequence homology with your protein and has the structure

$$R_1 — R_2 — R_3 — R_4 — R_5 — R_6 — R_7 — R_8$$

where R_8 is a full rather than a truncated repeat.

2. The protein product of the gene *STE4* in the yeast *Saccharomyces cerevisiae* has the following structure:

$$N — R_1 — R_2 — R_3 — R_4 — R_5 — R_6 — X — R_7 — R_8$$

where R_8 is a full rather than a truncated repeat.

3. The protein *groucho* from the fruit fly *Drosophila melanogaster*, coded for by a member of the gene complex *Enhancer of split* [*E(spl)*], has the following structure:

$$N - R_1 - R_2 - R_3 - R_4 - R_5 - X$$

Based on what is known or hypothesized about the functions of β-transducin, the *STE4* gene product and *groucho*, speculate about the possible normal role of the protein that is defective in your patient. Remember, you need to look up the functions of these proteins and then *speculate* about the possible role of your protein. The correct answer to this question is not yet known.

Answer 97

a. Cystatin C (MW 13,260) is an inhibitor of cysteine proteinases, a group of proteolytic enzymes that includes papain and the lysosomal cathepsins B, H, and L. Cystatic C, which occurs in the blood and elsewhere, is one of a group of small proteins that inhibit cysteine proteases; others in the group are cystatin A and cystatin B. These inhibitors may serve as regulators of the activities of these lysosomal proteases.

b. To figure out what happened to your patient, you need to line up the N-terminal sequences appropriately.

										Gly	Gly	Pro	Met	Asp	Ala	Ser	Val
Your patient:										Gly	Gly	Pro	Met	Asp	Ala	Ser	Val
Normal person:	Ser	Ser	Pro	Gly	Lys	Pro	Pro	Arg	Leu	Val	Gly	Gly	Pro	Met	Asp	Ala	Ser	Val

Clearly, your patient's cystatin C is missing the first 10 amino acids. There are three possible explanations: (1) the portion of the cystatin C gene coding for the N-terminal 10 amino acids has been deleted, (2) there is an alternative splicing mechanism going on which results in transcribing a mRNA missing the codons for the first 10 amino acids, or (3) there is altered posttranslational processing of your patient's cystatin C, causing cleavage of the first 10 amino acids. To decide between these two alternatives, look at what the two genes code for:

Codon number:	−26	−25	−24	−23		1	2	3	4		66	67	68	69	70
Your patient:															
DNA:	ATG	GCC	GGG	CCC	...	TCC	AGT	CCC	GGC	...	GTG	GAG	CAG	GGC	CGA
RNA:	AUG	GCC	GGG	CCC	...	UCC	AGU	CCC	GGC	...	GUG	GAG	CAG	GGC	CGA
Protein:	Met	Ala	Gly	Pro	...	Ser	Ser	Pro	Gly	...	Val	Glu	Gln	Gly	Arg
Normal person:															
DNA:	ATG	GCC	GGG	CCC	...	TCC	AGT	CCC	GGC	...	GTG	GAG	CTG	GGC	CGA
RNA:	AUG	GCC	GGG	CCC	...	UCC	AGU	CCC	GGC	...	GUG	GAG	CUG	GGC	CGA
Protein:	Met	Ala	Gly	Pro	...	Ser	Ser	Pro	Gly	...	Val	Glu	Leu	Gly	Arg

Cystatin C occurs in the blood in sufficient quantities for the altered protein to precipitate. As a secreted protein it must have a signal sequence. As you can deduce from the codon numbering as well as the hydrophobic nature of the four residues from −26 to −23, the signal sequence is present in your patient's cystatin C as well as in the normal cystatin C. The N-terminal region also appears to be present in your patient. Therefore, the first two possibilities must be eliminated. Your patient's gene and mRNA codes for the entire protein. In other words, her cystatin C is made with the first 10 amino acids, and the third possibility is correct. Your patient's cystatin C must be more susceptible to having its N-terminal region removed.

Notice the mutation at position 68. Your patient has a glutamine where a normal person has a leucine. This certainly alters the hydrophobicity at this spot. Also, there is a glycine at position 69 and the glutamine–glycine sequence has a high probability of forming a β-hairpin. Thus the mutation, although occurring distant from the N-terminal region, may make the cystatin C more susceptible to abnormal proteolysis. With the first 10 amino acids removed, the truncated cystatin C may have a tendency to aggregate. Aggregated cystatin C could clog blood vessels and lead to hemorrhage.

   c. Restriction endonucleases are enzymes that cleave DNA at specific sequences. They can be used for restriction mapping, in which the cleavage fragments are subjected to electrophoresis on a gel. AluI has the following specificity:

$$\downarrow$$
5'-A-G-C-T-3'   The arrows mark the points of cleavage by AluI.
3'-T-C-G-A-5'
$$\uparrow$$

If you look at the DNA sequence for codons 67 and 68 in a normal person, you will see the AGCT sequence:

        67   68
       GAG   CTG

Obviously, AluI could cleave at this point (between codons 67 and 68). In your patient, that sequence is altered:

        67   68
       GAG   CAG

AluI could not cleave here. Thus treatment of your patient's DNA with AluI would generate a different pattern of fragments than would treatment of normal DNA. Hence AluI could be a valuable diagnostic tool for looking for this particular mutation.

Your patient has HEREDITARY CYSTATIN C AMYLOID ANGIO-PATHY (HEREDITARY CEREBRAL HEMORRHAGE WITH AMYLOIDOSIS, ICELANDIC TYPE).

References

Barrett, A. J., Davies, M. E., and Grubb, A. The place of human γ-trace (cystatin C) amongst the cysteine proteinase inhibitors. *Biochem. Biophys. Res. Commun.* 120: 631, 1984.

Ghiso, J., Jensson, O., and Frangione, B. Amyloid fibrils in hereditary cerebral hemorrhage with amyloidosis of Icelandic type is a variant of γ-trace basic protein (cystatin C). *Proc. Natl. Acad. Sci. USA* 83: 2974, 1986.

Jensson, O., Palsdottir, A., Thorsteinsson, L., and Arnason, A. The saga of cystatin C mutation causing amyloid angiopathy and brain hemorrhage: clinical genetics in Iceland. *Clin. Genet.* 36: 368, 1989.

Jonsdottir, S., and Palsdottir, A. Molecular diagnosis of hereditary cystatin C amyloid angiopathy. *Biochem. Med. Metabol. Biol.* 49: 117, 1993.

Levy, E., Lopez-Otin, C., Ghiso, J., Geltner, D., and Frangione, B. Stroke in Icelandic patients with hereditary amyloid angiopathy is related to a mutation in the cystatin C gene, an inhibitor of cysteine proteases. *J. Exp. Med.* 169: 1771, 1989.

Roberts, R. J., Myers, P. A., Morrison, A., and Murray, K. A specific endonuclease from *Arthrobacter luteus*. *J. Mol. Biol.* 102: 157, 1976.

Sibanda, B. L., and Thornton, J. M. β-Hairpin families in globular proteins. *Nature* 316: 170, 1985.

Answer 98

a. First, convert the nucleotide sequence into an amino acid sequence:

Codon number:	1	2	3	4	5	...612	613	614	615	616	617	618	619	620	621	622	623	624
DNA:	ATG	CTG	CCC	GGT	TTG	...AAA	TTG	GTG	TTC	TTT	GCA	GAA	GAT	GTG	GGT	TCA	AAC	AAA
RNA:	AUG	CUG	CCC	GGU	UUG	...AAA	UUG	GUG	UUC	UUU	GCA	GAA	GAU	GUG	GGU	UCA	AAC	AAA
Protein:	Met	Leu	Pro	Gly	Leu	...Lys	Leu	Val	Phe	Phe	Ala	Glu	Asp	Val	Gly	Ser	Asn	Lys

Notice that the portion of your patient's peptide that you have sequenced lines up pretty well, but not perfectly, with a portion of the normal sequence of BAPP.

Codon number:	1	2	3	4	5	. . .	612	613	614	615	616	617	618	619	620	621	622	623	624
Protein:	Met	Leu	Pro	Gly	Leu	. . .	Lys	Leu	Val	Phe	Phe	Ala	Glu	Asp	Val	Gly	Ser	Asn	Lys
Peptide:						. . .	Lys	Leu	Val	Phe	Phe	Ala	Gln	Asp	Val	Gly	Ser	Asn	Lys

It appears likely that the peptide is a fragment of BAPP because the lineup is almost perfect. Presumably, therefore, the defect in your patient is that this peptide is cleaved from BAPP and then aggregates. Why exactly it is cleaved is not clear. Notice, however, the one residue where the two sequences do not match up. Position 618 in BAPP is glutamic acid where the corresponding position in the peptide is glutamine. Presumably your patient's BAPP has mutated to replace the glutamic acid at position 618 with a glutamine. Changing glutamic acid to glutamine could have two effects. First, it might alter the conformation of the BAPP protein and cause it to be cleaved at a place different from where it would normally be cleaved. The resulting 39-amino acid peptide is highly hydrophobic and likely to precipitate. Second, altering the glutamic acid to glutamine makes the peptide less charged and hence even more hydrophobic and increases the likelihood of precipitation. The precipitation then causes the peptide to accumulate and block the blood vessels, and this causes the hemorrhages.

b. MboII is a restriction endonuclease that cleaves DNA seven or eight nucleotides away from its recognition site:

$$\downarrow$$
5'-G-A-A-G-A-X-X-X-X-X-X-X-X-X-3'   The arrows mark the points of
3'-C-T-T-C-T-X-X-X-X-X-X-X-X-X-5'   cleavage by MboII.
$$\uparrow$$

You will notice that there is a recognition site in the DNA sequence corresponding to codons 618 and 619 in the gene for normal BAPP:

618   619
GAA   GAT

MboII would therefore cleave the DNA eight nucleotides downstream from this site. You do not know the mutated DNA sequence in your patient, but you know that it codes for glutamine instead of for glutamic acid. Therefore, the DNA sequence must be either

618	619	or	618	619
CAA	GAT		CAG	GAT

Neither of these contain the recognition site for *Mbo*II. Therefore, the site disappears in anyone who carries the mutated gene. A restriction map of this region of the DNA would therefore differ in these people from that of someone who has the normal gene.

Your patient has HEREDITARY CEREBRAL HEMORRHAGE, DUTCH TYPE.

References

Brown, N. L., Hutchison, C. A., and Smith, M. The specific nonsymmetrical sequence recognized by restriction endonuclease *Mbo*II. *J. Mol. Biol.* 140: 143, 1980.

Kang, J., Lemaire, H.-G., Unterbeck, A., Salbaum, J. M., Masters, C. L., Grzeschik, K.-H., Multhaup, G., Beyreuther, K., and Müller-Hill, B. The precursor of Alzheimer's disease amyloid A4 protein resembles a cell-surface receptor. *Nature* 325: 733, 1987.

Levy, E., Carman, M. D., Fernandez-Madrid, I. J., Power, M. D., Lieberburg, I., Van Duinen, S. G., Bots, G. T. A. M., Luyendijk, W., and Frangione, B. Mutation of the Alzheimer's disease amyloid gene in hereditary cerebral hemorrhage, Dutch type. *Science* 248: 1124, 1990.

Answer 99

a. This is apparently a problem of amyloidosis, of which there are several types. These are conditions where there is inappropriate cleavage of a protein, resulting in formation of a fragment that precipitates. The large protein is β-amyloid precursor protein (BAPP) and the small protein is amyloid β-protein (Aβ).

b. To understand this process better, you need to see the relevant portion of the sequence of BAPP:

Codon number:	589	590	591	592	593	594	595	596	597	598	599	600	601
Your patient:													
DNA:	GAG	GAG	ATC	TCT	GAA	GTG	AAT	CTG	GAT	GCA	GAA	TTC	CGA
RNA:	GAG	GAG	AUC	UCU	GAA	GUG	AAU	CUG	GAU	GCA	GAA	UUC	CGA
Protein:	Glu	Glu	Ilu	Ser	Glu	Val	Asn	Leu	Asp	Ala	Glu	Phe	Arg

Normal person:													
DNA:	GAG	GAG	ATC	TCT	GAA	GTG	AAG	ATG	GAT	GCA	GAA	TTC	CGA
RNA:	GAG	GAG	AUC	UCU	GAA	GUG	AAG	AUG	GAU	GCA	GAA	UUC	CGA
Protein:	Glu	Glu	Ilu	Ser	Glu	Val	Lys	Met	Asp	Ala	Glu	Phe	Arg

Your patient has an unusual mutation, a double transversion, in which a G has mutated to a T and the adjacent A to a C. These adjacent nucleotides occupy two codons, so two amino acids are altered; a Lys-Met becomes Asn-Leu. The significance of this becomes apparent when you line up the sequence near the mutation with the N-terminal sequence of the small protein that you isolated from your patient:

BAPP residue number:	589	590	591	592	593	594	595	596	597	598	599	600	601
BAPP:	Glu	Glu	Ilu	Ser	Glu	Val	Lys	Met	Asp	Ala	Glu	Phe	Arg
Aβ:									Asp	Ala	Glu	Phe	Arg
Aβ residue number:									1	2	3	4	5

We can conclude that when β-amyloid precursor protein is cleaved to generate the amyloid β-protein, the cleavage occurs between Met[596] and Asp[597]. The mutation may increase the cleavage, leading to production of more of the β-amyloid protein, which then would precipitate and impair nerve function.

Your patient has FAMILIAL ALZHEIMER'S DISEASE.

References

Citron, M., Oltersdorf, T., Haass, C., McConlogue, L., Hung, A. Y., Seubert, P., Vigo-Pelfrey, Lieberburg, I., and Selkoe, D. J. Mutation of the β-amyloid precursor protein in familial Alzheimer's disease increases β-protein production. *Nature* 360: 672, 1992.

Kang, J., Lemaire, H.-G., Unterbeck, A., Salbaum, J. M., Masters, C. L., Grzeschik, K.-H., Multhaup, G., Beyreuther, K. and Müller-Hill, B. The precursor of Alzheimer's disease amyloid A4 protein resembles a cell-surface receptor. *Nature* 325: 733, 1987.

Mullan, M., Crawford, F., Axelman, K., Houlden, H., Lilius, L., Winblad, B., and Lannfelt, L. A pathogenic mutation of probable Alzheimer's disease in the APP gene at the N-terminus of β-amyloid. *Nature Genet.* 1: 345, 1992.

Selkoe, D. J. The molecular pathology of Alzheimer's disease. *Neuron* 6: 487, 1991.

Seubert, P., Oltersdorf, T., Lee, M. K., Barbour, R., Blomquist, C., Davis, D. L., Bryant, K., Fritz, L. C., Galasko, D., Thal, L. J., Lieberburg, I., and Schenk, D. B. Secretion of β-amyloid precursor protein cleaved at the amino terminus of the β-amyloid peptide. *Nature* 361: 260, 1993.

Answer 100

Transducin is a 340-amino acid G protein involved in photoreception in the retina. Transducin has three subunits: α, β, and γ. When a photon of light hits the rhodopsin molecule, it induces a conformational change in rhodopsin, which in turn induces transducin to break up into an α subunit and the $\beta\gamma$ subunits (which remain together). The free α subunit then binds to and activates a phosphodiesterase that hydrolyzes cGMP. The lowered intracellular levels of cGMP then permit membrane Na^+ channels to be closed, and the subsequent hyperpolarization then causes a signal to be sent to the neurons of the optic nerve. The precise role of the β subunit is unclear, as is the case with the β subunits of many G proteins.

The product of the yeast gene *STE4* is also the β subunit (423 amino acids) of a G protein. This one is a protein that is involved in the mating of yeast cells. When yeast cells want to mate, they release pheromones. The pheromones bind to receptors on cells of the opposite mating type. These cells respond by activating certain genes and then by fusing with the cell of the opposite type. The pheromone receptor is a G protein. Disruption of the gene that codes for the α subunit causes the mating phenotype to be expressed all the time regardless of whether or not the pheromone is present. Disruption of the β subunit (which is encoded by the *STE4* gene) or the γ subunit prevents mating behavior. It would seem, therefore, that in this G protein, the α subunit plays an inhibitory role while the β or γ subunits activate the next molecule in this signaling pathway.

Groucho (719 amino acids) has some similarities in sequence to β-transducin. It is involved in development in the fruit fly *Drosophila*. At an early stage in development, certain cells in the neuroectoderm start to differentiate into neuroblasts, which then develop into the central nervous system. Neuroectoderm cells that do not develop into neuroblasts go on to become either glia or epidermal cells. *Groucho* is one of several proteins that are involved in the determination of the fate of these cells, whether they will become neuroblasts or epidermal cells. Mutants lacking a functional *groucho* protein exhibit hypertrophy of the nervous system and loss of certain epidermal structures. Some mutants of *groucho* have duplicated head bristles. The *Enhancer of split* gene locus also contains genes for several other proteins, four of which have sequences resembling those of DNA-binding proteins.

Your protein resembles the β subunit of two known G proteins (β-transducin and the *STE4* gene product) and one probable G protein (*groucho*). It is therefore very likely that your protein is also the β subunit of a G protein. G proteins are generally associated with receptors, as is the case with the *STE4* gene product. The normal pattern is that when an activator, such as a hormone, binds to the receptor, the latter undergoes a conformational change which is transmitted to the G protein. The effect on the G protein is that the α subunit (G_α) detaches from the β and γ subunits ($G_{\beta\gamma}$) and, carrying its bound GTP, becomes associated with an enzyme that will activate the "second messenger." Such an enzyme might be adenyl cyclase, which makes cAMP. A variety of other proteins are involved. In some cases the G_α subunit plays an inhibitory role. Recent evidence suggests that the $G_{\beta\gamma}$ subunit may also play a signaling role in certain cases. It is likely, however, that your protein is part of a G protein associated with a receptor.

What would this receptor be? This is hard to say, but it is interesting that both the *STE4* gene product and *groucho* are involved in differentiation. The *STE4* gene product causes a yeast cell to acquire a mating morphology. *Groucho* causes neuroectodermal cells in *Drosophila* to become epidermal structures. Probably, your protein is a receptor for a growth factor acting early in embryonic life.

With which proteins might your protein interact? This is a very difficult question to answer in our present state of knowledge. Is it just a coincidence that mutations in both *groucho* and your protein affect development of both the central nervous system and the head? Perhaps your protein transmits a signal that activates or inactivates a protein which binds to DNA to induce or repress expression of genes involved in determining the differentiation of certain cells that will give rise to the brain and other parts of the head.

Your patient has MILLER–DIEKER LISSENCEPHALY.

References

Artavanis-Tsakonas, S., Delidakis, C., and Fehon, R. G. The *Notch* and the cell biology of neuroblast segregation. *Annu. Rev. Cell Biol.* 7: 427, 1991.

Cabrera, C. V. The generation of cell diversity during early neurogenesis in *Drosophila*. *Development* 115: 893, 1992.

Campos-Ortega, J. A., and Jan, Y. N. Genetic and molecular bases of neurogenesis in *Drosophila melanogaster*. *Annu. Rev. Neurosci.* 14: 399, 1991.

Dobyns, W. B. The neurogenetics of lissencephaly. *Neurol. Clin.* 7: 89, 1989.

Hartley, D. A., Preiss, A., and Artavanis-Tsakonas, S. A deduced gene product from the *Drosophila* neurogenic locus, *Enhancer of split,* shows homology to mammalian G-protein β subunit. *Cell* 55: 785, 1988.

Klämbt, C., Knust, E., Tietze, K., and Campos-Ortega, J. A. Closely related transcripts encoded by the neurogenic gene complex Enhancer of split of *Drosophila melanogaster.* *EMBO J.* 8: 203, 1989.

Leberer, E., Dignard, D., Hougan, L., Thomas, D. Y., and Whiteway, M. Dominant-negative mutants of a yeast G-protein β subunit identify two functional regions involved in pheromone signaling. *EMBO J.* 11: 4805, 1992.

Ledbetter, S. A., Kuwano, A., Dobyns, W. B., and Ledbetter, D. H. Microdeletions of chromosome 17p13 as a cause of isolated lissencephaly. *Am. J. Hum. Genet.* 50: 182, 1992.

Miller, J. Q. Lissencephaly in 2 siblings. *Neurology* 13: 841, 1963.

Preiss, A., Hartley, D. A., and Artavanis-Tsakonas, S. The molecular genetics of *Enhancer of split,* a gene required for embryonic neural development in *Drosophila.* *EMBO J.* 7: 3917, 1988.

Reiner, O., Carrozzo, R., Shen, Y., Wehnert, M., Faustinella, F., Dobyns, W. B., Caskey, C. T., and Ledbetter, D. H. Isolation of a Miller–Dieker lissencephaly gene containing G protein β-subunit-like repeats. *Nature* 364: 717, 1993.

Stryer, L. *Biochemistry.* New York: W.H. Freeman and Company, 1988, pp. 1033–1034.

Index